ETHICS AND PSYCHIATRY: TOWARD PROFESSIONAL DEFINITION

ETHICS AND PSYCHIATRY: TOWARD PROFESSIONAL DEFINITION

Allen R. Dyer, M.D., Ph.D.

PROFESSOR AND ASSOCIATE CHAIRMAN
DEPARTMENT OF PSYCHIATRY
THE ALBANY MEDICAL COLLEGE

CHIEF MEDICAL OFFICER
CAPITAL DISTRICT PSYCHIATRIC CENTER
ALBANY, NEW YORK

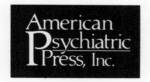

1400 K Street, N.W.
Washington, DC 20005

Books published by the American Psychiatric Press, Inc., represent the views and opinions of the individual authors and do not necessarily represent the policies and opinions of the Press or the American Psychiatric Association.

Library of Congress Cataloging-in-Publication Data

Dyer, Allen R.
    Ethics and psychiatry

    Bibliography: p.
    Includes index.
    1. Psychiatric ethics. I. Title [DNLM: 1. Ethics, Medical. 2. Psychiatry.
WM 62 D996e]
RC 455.2.E8D94   1987   174.2   87-1337
ISBN 0-88048-225-7

·CONTENTS·

Preface   *ix*

INTRODUCTION: A DIVIDED PROFESSION   *1*

  A DIVIDED PROFESSION
  THE MORAL PROBLEM OF OUR TIME
  THE DE-PROFESSIONALIZATION OF MEDICINE
  THE END OF HIPPOCRATIC MEDICINE?
  PSYCHIATRY AND THE MEDICAL MODEL
  THE PROGRAM OF THIS TEXT

·1· *THE PLACE OF ETHICS IN THE DEFINITION
     OF A PROFESSION*   *15*

  THE DEFINITION OF A PROFESSION
  THE SOCIOLOGY OF PROFESSIONS
  PROFESSION AND MONOPOLY
  THE ANTITRUST CHALLENGE TO THE
      PROFESSIONS
  THE ETHICS OF ADVERTISING
  CONCLUSION
  APPENDIX 1   American Medical Association
      Principles of Medical Ethics

·2· *THE HIPPOCRATIC TRADITION IN
     MEDICINE AND PSYCHIATRY*   *29*

  THE HIPPOCRATIC OATH
      Patient Confidentiality
      Abortion
      Euthanasia

Truth-Telling
Sexual Contact with Patients
Professional Affiliations
Justice in the Distribution of Health Services
Patient Benefit
THE CASE AGAINST HIPPOCRATIC MEDICINE
The Hippocratic Oath Is Anachronistic
The Hippocratic Oath Doesn't Deal with the
Highest Ethical Obligations of the Physician
The Hippocratic Oath Opposes Abortion and
Euthanasia
Hippocratic Medicine Has Been Faulted for
Defining Medical Care Mainly in Terms of
Emergency Treatment
The Patient Benefit Principle of the Hippocratic
Writings is Paternalistic
IN DEFENSE OF THE HIPPOCRATIC TRADITION
CONFLICTING DEMANDS UPON THE PHYSICIAN
Cooperation with Torture
Political Abuse of Psychiatry
Lethal Injections in Capital Punishment
Cost Containment
SUMMARY
APPENDIX 1   OATH OF HIPPOCRATES
APPENDIX 2   HIPPOCRATIC OATH FOR
PSYCHIATRISTS

·3· *THE TASKS AND METHODS OF ETHICS*   **45**

WHAT IS ETHICS? MEDICAL ETHICS?
Teleological Ethical Theories
Deontological Ethical Theories
The Consequentialist Approach

·4· *CONFIDENTIALITY, TRUST, AND THE*
THERAPEUTIC ALLIANCE   **59**

THE NEED FOR CONFIDENTIALITY
THREATS TO CONFIDENTIALITY
The *Tarasoff* Case: Protecting Public Safety
Preventing Fraud: Review of Medicare Records
Redisclosure in Information Banks
Cost Containment and Using the Physician as
an Agent of Rationing Health Care

Prearraignment Examinations
Advancing Scientific Knowledge: Case Reports
Professional Gossip
Access to Records by Patients
Treating the Same Person in Both Individual
    and Group Therapy
Psychiatric Testimony in Custody Cases
Nonprofessionals on Health Care Teams
Mandatory Reporting of Suspected Child Abuse
THE DOUBLE AGENT PROBLEM
LEGAL PERSPECTIVES ON THE ETHICAL
    PRINCIPLE

·5·   *A CRITIQUE OF SZASZ'S CRITIQUE: THE*
MIND-BODY PROBLEM WON'T GO AWAY   **71**

THE LEGACY OF CARTESIAN DUALISM
THE DEFINITION OF MEDICINE
THE "MYTH" OF MENTAL ILLNESS
UNDERSTANDING HYSTERIA
INVOLUNTARY HOSPITALIZATION
THE ETHICS OF GIVING PLACEBOS
THE DIFFERENCE BETWEEN PLACEBOS AND THE
    PLACEBO EFFECT

·6·   *INFORMED CONSENT, AUTONOMY, AND*
PATERNALISM: RESPECTING THE PATIENT IN
RESEARCH AND PRACTICE   **83**

THE PRINCIPLE OF AUTONOMY
THE ASSESSMENT OF COMPETENCE
TOWARD A DEFINITION OF INFORMED
    CONSENT
THE PRINCIPLE OF PARTNERSHIP
BEYOND THE IMPASSE
INFORMED CONSENT IN GREAT BRITAIN
INFORMED CONSENT IN SWEDEN
INFORMED CONSENT IN JAPAN AND THE ASIAN
    PACIFIC
INFORMED CONSENT BEHIND THE IRON
    CURTAIN
INFORMED CONSENT AND TORTURE
CONCLUSION

•7• *THE PLACE OF VIRTUE AND CHARACTER IN ETHICS: PSYCHIATRY'S CONTRIBUTION TO ETHICS*   *99*

    MORAL AND THERAPEUTIC CONSIDERATIONS
       OF CHARACTER
    CHARACTER AS CHARACTERISTIC
    CHARACTER AS RESISTANCE
    DEVELOPMENT OF THE PSYCHOANALYTIC
       THEORY OF CHARACTER
    CHARACTER AND MORAL DEVELOPMENT
    THE PSYCHOANALYTIC TREATMENT OF
       CHARACTER DISORDERS
    THE IMPORTANCE OF VIRTUE IN PROFESSIONAL
       GATEKEEPING
    THE CENTRAL VIRTUES OF THE MEDICAL
       PROFESSION
    THE VIRTUES OF THE PATIENT
    CONCLUSION

•8• *IDEALISM IN MEDICAL ETHICS: THE PURSUIT OF MORAL PERFECTION*   *111*

    THE SELF AS MORAL AGENT
    THE CONTEXT OF ETHICAL DECISION MAKING
    PERSONHOOD
    THE CRISIS OF THE PERSONAL
    THE MORAL SELF
    SHAME AND GUILT AS REGULATORS OF
       MORALITY
    THE PROBLEM OF THE MORAL INVERSION
    CONCLUSIONS

•9• *THE IMPEACHMENT OF ALTRUISM*   *129*

•10• *THE MEANING OF MEDICAL RESPONSIBILITY*   *137*

ENDNOTES   *149*

BIBLIOGRAPHY   *161*

INDEX   *169*

PREFACE

THIS BOOK IS DEDICATED to William H. Poteat. In the year of his retirement, this is but one of several books his students are giving back to him. Poteat, as he is fondly known, has taught a generation of college professors to think "post-critically" and to teach their students to do the same. In over three decades of teaching at Duke, he directed literally dozens of Ph.D. dissertations and taught thousands of students through a unique kind of classroom colloquy in which they learned not only to discern patterns of thought but, even more important, to articulate accounts of themselves, their views, their values, and their commitments.

Since this book is so thoroughly informed by the post-critical enterprise, it is worth offering a few words of orientation at the outset. The post-critical project was envisioned by Michael Polanyi in a series of books including *Science, Faith and Society, Personal Knowledge,* and *The Tacit Dimension.* Polanyi was concerned that claims of objectivity in knowing falsified knowledge and obscured the human values involved in believing something to be true. Science could not be value-neutral, but people could pretend not to be committed to the beliefs they held. Polanyi, who was trained as a physical chemist and made innovative discoveries in the field of crystallography (some of which challenged previously established beliefs), spoke of the inescapable tacit dimension involved in coming to know something. "We know more than we can tell," he reminded us, "but we can tell nothing without relying on our awareness of things we may not be able to tell" (Personal Knowledge, p. x).

Polanyi is thus a bit like the child in the story of the emperor's new clothes. He reminds us what we already know but are afraid to acknowledge. The ideal of strict objectivism is absurd. Any particular commitment can be challenged but only on the grounds of a rival commitment. The life of the scientific community consists of enforcing the tradition of science and assuring at the same time its continuous renewal. This requires a dynamic and free society, not rigid or authoritarian dogmatism. Science requires an affirmation of belief. If this requirement is not acknowledged, rigid dogmatism can result. This rigidity undermines any validity objectivism might claim.

In illustrating the structure of tacit knowing, Polanyi draws on two distinctions that are informative of the problems faced in modern medicine and medical ethics. He distinguishes tacit and explicit knowledge and focal and subsidiary awareness. When we drive a nail with a hammer, we are focally aware of the movements of the hammer, but only subsidiarily aware of the position of the hammer in our hand. These two kinds of awareness are mutually exclusive. If we shift our awareness to our hand on the hammer, we become clumsy in the execution of our task.

Similarly the practice of medicine relies on acts of judgment that cannot be completely specified. Just as one could not give a sufficient description of a stranger to be met at an airport, so a skilled clinician could not give an abstract account of the factors involved in making a diagnosis or deciding on a wise course of treatment. Similarly the responsible decisions of the ethical clinician cannot be abstracted into a list of rules. Any attempts at abstract analysis of ethical quandaries potentially make us awkward in the practice of medicine when attending to the needs of a particular patient.

These observations may well remind the psychiatrist of the importance of attending to unconscious motivations as well as overt behavior. While Polanyi himself was concerned with Freud's reliance on mechanistic and electrodynamic metaphors for human experience, the enterprise of psychoanalysis and the post-critical enterprise both share much in common in the emphasis on the importance of self-knowledge and acknowledgment of one's moral commitments in relationship to others in society. This emphasis recalls the ambitions of ancient philosophers to "know thyself," as the Socratic admonition put it. It also recalls the importance of communication with others in what Polanyi would call a "convivial order": in the colloquies of Poteat's classroom, free associations on the psychoanalyst's couch, or in derivative forms of psychotherapy.

Philosophers often make a point of stressing that ethics is not psychotherapy. The task of ethics, they argue, is to clarify moral dilemmas and to provide a rational basis for deciding among competing theories. This view of ethics rests on the epistemological assumption, prevalent in the modern world, that knowledge is based on objective and explicitly verifiable units that can be rationally determined. While this is a laudable concept, psychiatrists—and many moral philosophers as well—recognize the irrational antecedents of adult rationality. Ethical theory must deal not only with the search for wisdom but also with the question of virtue. Wisdom is knowing what to do next, as one aphorism puts it, and virtue is doing it. Ethics, like psychotherapy, can help a person to better understand himself or herself in relation to the decisions being faced.

It is my ambition in this book not so much to settle the various controversies surrounding medicine and psychiatry by persuading the reader of the wisdom of my own views as it is to provide an intellectual framework of these controversies for intelligent debate in which the responsible individual may find his or her own commitments.

I am very grateful to a number of colleagues who have read the manuscript in various forms of revision along the way and have offered comments that have helped shape its development: Larry Churchill, who reassured me that the book is complicated because there are no simple solutions for complicated problems, Doug Adams, Stanley Hauerwas, Ylanna Miller, Alan Stern, William Webb, Ewald Busse, and Robert Moore. My students have thoughtfully reflected on the manuscript in light of their concerns in becoming physicians. My secretary, Connie Rayborn, master of the new technology, has carefully edited, referenced, and indexed. She has been assisted by William Saunders in Duke's psychiatry research support office. My wife, Susan, who has followed my work through eighteen years of marriage and longer, has offered loving encouragement, pleasant diversions, incisive comments, and inspiration.

I would also like to acknowledge a number of foundations that have supported my work over the past decade. They have become partners in the enterprise, and I would never have been able to pursue graduate study in religion and medical ethics along with a medical career if it had not been for their support at crucial points along the way. They have all contributed to work reflected in this book in various ways. The Danforth Foundation provided a Kent Fellowship, which paid for graduate school tuition. The Institute for Human Values in Medicine provided a fellowship for dissertation research. The National Fund for Medical Education provided a fellowship, which supported me during the year of writing the Ph.D. dissertation, as well as grants to teach cost containment issues in medical ethics and to investigate the application of moral development theory to the medical school admissions process. The Hunt Foundation and Roy A. Hunt Foundation of Pittsburgh provided a series of grants that supported the teaching of medical ethics at Duke University Medical Center over a five-year period. The W. K. Kellogg Foundation awarded me a Kellogg National Fellowship, which brought me into regular contact with a network of some of the most stimulating people I have ever met and provided me with an awareness of global interdependence. It also enabled me to undertake a cross-national study of the teaching of medical ethics and regulation of the medical professions, which involved meeting colleagues in Great Britain, Belgium, West Germany, Sweden, Austria, Yugoslavia, France, Brazil, India, Thailand, Hong Kong, and Japan. The Josiah Charles Trent Memorial Foundation also contributed to this study. The National Humanities Center provided me with another fellowship that offered time to begin my studies of professional definition and offered a most convivial setting. The Department of Psychiatry at the University of Oxford provided me with an academic home for a sabbatical year and a return visit during which most of this book was written.

I would like to add one other acknowledgment: to my first teacher of what it means to be a professional, my father. I remember one of his patients telling me that when she was in his office, she felt like she was the only person in the world. If we can succeed in passing this legacy of patient-centered attentiveness on to our own patients, our children, and our students, then the professions may not be in such precarious condition.

Some of the ideas presented in this book have been reworked from earlier publications:

My Ph.D. dissertation, "Idealism in Medical Ethics: The Problem of the Moral Inversion," deals much more extensively with the issues addressed in Chapter 8 and with the implications of Michael Polanyi's epistemology for ethics and medical ethics. It is available from University Microfilms (Ann Arbor, Michigan) in microfilm or printed hardcopy.

Following are references for papers related to parts of chapters of this book:

Ethics, advertising, and the definition of a profession, *Journal of Medical Ethics* 11:72-78, 1985.

Can informed consent be obtained from a psychiatric patient? Reflections on the doctor-patient relationship, in *Controversy in Psychiatry*. Edited by John Paul Brady and H. Keith H. Brodie. Philadelphia: Saunders, 1978, pp. 983-996.

Informed consent and the psychiatric patient, with Sidney Bloch. *Journal of Medical Ethics* 13:12–16,1987.

Informed consent and the non-autonomous person. *IRB: A Review of Human Subjects Research*, a publication of The Hastings Center 5(7):1–4 August-September 1982.

Assessment of competence to give informed consent, in *Senile Dementias of the Alzheimer's Type and Related Diseases: Ethical and Legal Issues Related to Informed Consent*. Edited by Vijaya L. Melnick. Clifton, NJ: Humana Press, 1985.

Virtue and medicine: a physician's analysis, in *Virtue and Medicine*. Edited by Earl Shelp. Dordrecht: D. Reidel, 1985, pp. 223-235.

The concept of character: moral and therapeutic considerations. *British Journal of Medical Psychology*, 59:35-41, March 1986.

INTRODUCTION

A DIVIDED PROFESSION

WE TURN TO ETHICS in times of crisis or uncertainty in hopes of resolving conflicts in a civil and reflective manner. Recent years have witnessed unprecedented interest in medical ethics, reflecting the crisis and uncertainty surrounding the medical profession. Something is wrong; everyone knows it. Technology is usually blamed. Ethical discussion often focuses on the headline controversies about how to apply wisely the latest technologies relating to artificial organs, baboon-to-human transplants, or in vitro fertilization, or how to deal with those who might not want all this technology.

Less attention has been given to the day-to-day issues of practice, which were once the main substance of medical ethics and which might provide a human context for assessing the application of technology. Medical practice has in some very serious ways been divorced from its ethical traditions so that it becomes possible to imagine medicine as merely technology and physicians as merely technicians. The old rhetoric about the ethics of the doctor-patient relationship seems quaint as we are confronted with an impersonal new technology. Medical ethics has largely become the ethics of strangers, with the doctor and patient not known to each other as persons. Yet the prodigious success of "scientific medicine" has raised a curious paradox: Though it is possible for the new technology to be applied in an impersonal manner, more is required of medicine in meeting human needs.

A DIVIDED PROFESSION

Psychiatry as part of medicine is caught up in the vortex of society rethinking the new technologies and the meaning of professional relationships. Psychiatry as part of medicine is heir to the long ethical traditions of professional

1

identity, and as part of medicine, psychiatry is a beneficiary of many of the new technologies. Yet psychiatry is a divided profession. It is divided by competing definitions of both "profession" and "medical." While there are many different persuasions in psychiatry, the most obvious split is that between the "biological" and "psychological." Those who practice biological psychiatry identify themselves closely with medicine and see psychiatry as treatment of physical disorders. Those in the psychological camp may be of a number of different persuasions emphasizing the learned determinants of behavior, the social elements, or the developmental intrapsychic nature of emotional conflict. At its best psychiatry is a profession representing a mosaic of orientations, an integration of the knowledge of many disciplines. At its worst it may seem hopelessly fragmented.

The skills a successful psychiatrist must master are diverse indeed, and some degree of specialization is inevitably necessary. But integration of diverse approaches is really the keystone of successful practice. Lest one attempt to fit the patient into a "Procrustean couch" of the doctor's favorite treatment, one must first assess the needs of a particular patient in light of the treatment options available. It is the assessment of the patient's problems with compassionate humane understanding in light of good scientific evidence that characterizes the medical model more than does allegiance to one camp or another.

But what is humane understanding and what is scientific evidence? These larger questions suggest that it would be useful to consider psychiatry as a prototypical profession. The whole range of ethical questions in medicine—from birth to death, abortion to euthanasia—hinge on what we mean by humane understanding and scientific evidence. Is medicine merely the application of biological science to human problems, or does the physician's healing art go deeper? Is the current widespread dissatisfaction with the medical profession caused by a too-narrow application of technique, a "treat-the-disease-and-forget-the-person" approach? If so, psychiatry should not look to medicine for its professional identity—at least it should not look to a reductionistic view of medicine. Rather, psychiatry should instruct medicine by its attempts to integrate complex understanding of diverse facts and theories in the service of the patient's needs.

This is not just a book about ethics for psychiatrists. It is a book about ethics for all professionals and all those interested in the ethical problems posed by professional life. It focuses on psychiatry not just for the interesting ethical dilemmas that occur in psychiatric practice, but for the way in which psychiatric insight illuminates professional activity. Psychiatry is viewed here as the quintessential profession. In no other profession does the relationship between the professional and the person served receive such scrutiny. It is the ethics of that personal relationship of service as much as the knowledge of the practitioner that defines a profession and distinguishes a profession from a trade.

THE MORAL PROBLEM OF OUR TIME

Two very different approaches to ethics have emerged partly as a response to the stunning perplexities of modern technology. One might be characterized as "quandary ethics."[1] The approach of quandary ethics is to analyze the dilemmas presented by such situations as the emergence of artificial organs or in vitro fertilization in hopes of coming up with some appropriate social policy for dealing with them. The other approach, which may be called "character ethics," asks very different sorts of questions; namely, "What sort of person do I wish to become?" and more broadly "What sort of society do we collectively wish to become by the choices we make?"[2] Inevitably the methods of the two approaches are very different, but even more important is the tension between the two approaches as modes of thought.

Quandary ethics aspires to be impersonal, even objective, and hopes to settle issues in a manner which transcends time, history, culture, and person. Universality is the stated ambition of quandary analysis. This approach is often contemptuous of the kind of ambiguities that must necessarily attend reflections on character, culture, and personality. Character ethics is the background against which we see our quandaries. If we focus on the quandary, we may become awkward in the execution of our responsibilities. Either reflection on character or quandary is awkward and incomplete in itself. Doug Adams and Phil Mullins, demonstrating that "human knowing is a moral enterprise guided by conscience," show how both approaches are necessary.[3] They exist in a proximal-distal relationship. The resolution of quandaries is the location for the actions of the moral self.

The tension between objectivity and subjectivity pervades ethical reflection in medicine as it has the reflections on knowing and doing ever since the Enlightenment philosophers of the seventeenth and eighteenth centuries established the ideal of "objectivity" as the only valid form of knowing. Descartes described a "method" of systematic doubting as the way of establishing knowledge, unreflective of the person doing the doubting.[4] Bacon described the scientific method in terms of observation and experimentation without any systematic reflection on the goals or purposes of the phenomenon to be understood. Thus "facts" and "values" came to exist as two separate realms of knowledge. Part of the tension in medicine stems from a "two cultures" dichotomy that has persisted in Western society since the Enlightenment, in which there is open conflict between the commitments of the "sciences" camp, with an emphasis on objectivity, fact, abstraction, and certainty, and the cause of the "humanities," with an emphasis on subjectivity, value, emotion, and experience.

The pronouncement of C. P. Snow—that the sciences and the humanities have come to represent two cultures that have so little in common that they never meet—has been widely accepted. Yet this conclusion must ultimately be unacceptable for modern medicine. Is Snow right? Or is Michael Polanyi right when he suggests that because of the unspecifiable elements in the human process of scientific discovery, the objectivist account of knowing is false, and "Science, conceived as understanding nature, seamlessly joins with the humanities, bent on the understanding of man and human greatness."[5]

Medicine has seemed in many ways to be the fulfillment of the Enlightenment promise of a better world through control of nature, but this ambition is acquired at high human cost. What ends should technology serve? The question cannot be answered impersonally. Ideally the profession of medicine should be in a good position to bridge the cultural gap between the sciences and the humanities with its dual epistemological heritage, the art and science of medicine. However, both medical practitioners and the public have been led to misperceive the nature and larger human setting of medical technology, to misvalue it and thus to be led by it to grandiose expectations. The result is a highly technological approach to medical practice. In spite of this, medicine is more than just medical technology.

It is an interesting footnote on history that the false ideals of objective knowledge have largely been discredited by philosophers and physical scientists while still largely held to by medical and behavioral scientists. Physicists recognized that they could not measure both the position and velocity of very small particles without their participation affecting the outcome of the measurement, the so-called "Heisenberg Uncertainty Principle." Thus it was recognized that the most precise of sciences, like all human activities, required judgments of determination. This is a striking analogy for psychiatric practice —and all of medical practice as well—in which the outcome of any investigation is greatly influenced by the participation of the observer, or conversely by the absence of the participation of the physician/scientist.

Polanyi has observed that the ideal of scientific detachment is perhaps harmless in the exact sciences, for it is in fact disregarded there by scientists. But, he observes, it exercises a destructive influence in biology, psychology, and sociology and falsifies our whole outlook far beyond the domain of science.[6] The destructive influence of which he speaks is the uncoupling of valuing and knowing that occurs when we do not acknowledge the value components of that which we claim to know. This point might be beyond our present concerns but for a similar uncoupling of valuing and knowing in the professions and professional ethics.

THE DE-PROFESSIONALIZATION OF MEDICINE

As we ask what defines a profession, we find that the same false dichotomy between the sciences and the humanities has found its way into the popular imagination concerning the professions. The two dominant and competing views of what defines a profession are that a profession is defined by (1) the knowledge or technical expertise of the professional, or (2) the ethics of the professional group, specifically the fiduciary commitments of the doctor-patient (or professional-client) relationship, commitments based on trust.

The distinction between knowledge (or expertise) and ethics might once have been unthinkable. Knowledge was a very personal thing and could not be separated from the values of the knower or user of the knowledge. But scientific medicine has been so successful on a reductionistic model—treating the patient as a thing to be manipulated—that it becomes much easier to uncouple expertise and ethics. Indeed it becomes much easier to imagine medicine as merely the application of technology and to view service as a commodity and a profession as a business.

Ethics in such a view no longer pervade the character of professional and civic life, but represent another technique of analysis to be invoked at extreme moments for high-technology dilemmas or quandaries.

Even the phrase "medical ethics" is passing from currency in recent years, being replaced by "biomedical ethics" and more recently by "bioethics." This movement may be taken on the one hand as recognition that the problems seen a decade ago as medical problems (and which have been seen as matters of physician discretion) really involve the most fundamental values of society, not just the concerns of physicians and patients. The elimination of a medical focus may also represent a shift of confidence, an erosion of public trust in the medical profession, perhaps even a sense that the physician has become merely a technician, or as economic jargon becomes more pervasive, merely a "provider."

Explicit attention to ethics might be seen as a corrective humanizing force in medical education. In fact, however, medical ethics and bioethics often have their own paradoxically dehumanizing effect on medical practice. By removing ethical reflection from the clinical arena to the arena of public policy and attempting to establish ethics as a rival rather than a coordinate discipline, one in which the physician is said to have little "expertise," even thinking about ethics is estranged from actual decision making.

The irony of this development lies in its circularity. The charge that can legitimately be leveled against the technocrat is that of shortsightedness, in which decisions are based on private judgment, unconscious of value conflicts. The ethicist may rightly repudiate this arrogation of power, but cannot at the same time claim to be the true expert in ethical reasoning. It is often true that physicians are poorly trained in ethics and may assume that the warrants of their judgments lie in their special training or "expertise." As unfortunate as this misunderstanding may be philosophically, it is largely mitigated by the personal concern most physicians still demonstrate for their patients; however, the same arrogance in a philosopher may have devastating consequences. Physicians and philosophers may thus seem naive to each other: physicians for deciding with a paucity of ethical reflection, philosophers for arguing at a level of abstraction or criticism so far removed from the complexity of real-life situations as to appear ultimately hollow.[7]

Here is a brief but sobering example of this challenge to medicine, played out so many ways in the "who decides?" discussions. A prominent ethicist seeking experience in medicine went onto an orthopedics ward and asked the residents if they had any ethical problems. Thinking he meant terminal patients on respirators or some of the usual headline issues often spoken of as ethical dilemmas, the residents replied that they currently had no ethical problems. He then examined the charts of two patients with similar fractures and found that one patient had received Demerol for pain and the other had received only Darvon. He then concluded that these were not medical decisions but ethical decisions *instead*.[8]

The physicians acted on their values unreflectively; the philosopher abstracted ethical reflection from the context in which an action was to be taken. In attempting to demonstrate the centrality of ethics in clinical judgment, he regrettably separated thought from action. A valid point could be made that choice of analgesic involves human values, attitudes toward pain and suffering, and compassion for the patient. To say that these concerns are not medical reinforces the prejudice that medicine is merely a technical enterprise and further implies that a physician may or must defer ethical reflection to a specialist in ethics. This view is nothing short of scandalous and literally depersonalizes both reflection on the practice of medicine and reflection on ethics as well. Indeed a cogent case could be made for saying that physicians do not need detached analysis of ethical "problems"; they need instead to be shown how to appreciate and accredit their own personal, humane judgment. "Clinical judgment" very much involves ethical choices even in mundane examples. This is an important realization in medical education because there is a real tendency for medical students and physicians, confronted by their hostile critics, to attempt the impossible: to limit their concern to technical matters, which can be carefully defended.

The need for a reaffirmation that the individual is responsible for his or her actions should be obvious to anyone reflecting on ethics and might even seem trivial were it not for the devastating credibility we have come unreflectively to accord to the demands of objectivity. We have come so thoroughly to expect an exhaustive and explicit account of behavior (we once might have said "conduct") that we become suspicious of any attempts to wrestle with the personal ambiguities involved in the decision-making process. When an ethicist such as Robert Veatch argues that physicians have little training in ethics, but are deeply involved in making ethical decisions, we are easily led to his conclusion that this is a "generalization of expertise," the translation of expertise from a technical area to a moral area.[9] We are too ready to accept that the physician should refrain from making moral judgments because we accept the specialization of forms of knowing and accept that there could be such a thing as a value-free technical judgment independent of moral considerations. Physicians and nonphysicians alike participate in this *folie à deux* because it is part of our common cultural heritage. We ask for a precise clarification of issues when we know that is not possible. Yet neither physician nor patient would dare say very much about the personal commitments that might bear on a particular decision when such personal disclosure might be subject to critical scrutiny.

Thus matters of personal ethics very quickly get translated into matters of public policy. We are relatively more comfortable analyzing issues than we are in looking at ourselves and our conflicted motives for action. Medical ethics provide a fruitful area for investigation since the decisions of the physician are of such obvious consequence, but self-scrutiny for the physician may be particularly difficult because the physician's decisions are made so publicly and because they are so often made in the company of strangers. We should not conclude, however, that because the decisions of the physician are of such obvious consequence, they are inherently different from the decisions of any other citizens in our culture. All involve the living of lives, the making of choices, and the interaction of individuals with others who may not share our commitments and values.

Our culture inhibits moral reflection at a personal level. It encourages us to alienate our moral authority to an expert or system of rules. In a culture both skeptical and (morally) perfectionistic, ideals are confused with imperatives. Legitimate moral ideals are not recognized as goals toward which one might strive, but rather are held as imperatives to which one must adhere.

If it can be credibly claimed that ethics is a matter of "expertise" in which one can be cognitively trained, then a profession can be conceived of independently of the ethics of its members. If a profession is nothing but technical expertise, then it might as well be regulated merely as a trade, an "industry" in the marketplace.

This impersonal view of ethics is firmly established and probably explains why ethical alarm bells were not sounded when the Federal Trade Commission (FTC) filed suit against the American Medical Association (AMA) in 1975, holding that the AMA was in restraint of trade under the Sherman Antitrust Act because its code of ethics prohibited advertising. The FTC eventually won its case, and the decision by the Supreme Court in 1983 held that the AMA could not have a code of ethics unless approved first by the Federal Trade Commission.

The legal issues here are complex and will be dealt with in greater detail in Chapter 1. However, the crucial point is that the uncoupling of ethics and expertise has become so much a feature of modern culture that the FTC's action was accepted with little protest. It has become customary to consider a profession as largely technical and to consider ethics as an impersonal analysis of quandaries. Medicine in fact is no longer considered or treated as a profession; it is conceived largely as a technology. Thus it is considered appropriate for medicine to be regulated, the same as any impersonal business. The binding strictures of professional ethics, not just the written codes of ethics but the more tacit interpersonal "covenants," are replaced by the suspicions of the marketplace: *Caveat emptor*, Let the Buyer Beware. The burdens of responsibility are shifted from the professional to what we now regularly refer to as the "consumer," professional care having become along the way a "commodity."

I hope that many will recoil at the prospect of this split between ethics and expertise. I hope that many physicians will insist that ethics is very much a part of their professional lives and their personal identities as physicians. I hope that by looking at the question of professional definition, we will realize that there is much to be lost by accepting the standards of the marketplace, the laws of supply and demand, or even the kind of moral rules that can be made completely explicit. Ultimately, however imperfect their demands, the human imperatives of trust and good faith must guide the conscientious physician to standards higher than those that can be explicitly specified.

THE END OF HIPPOCRATIC MEDICINE?

The Hippocratic Oath is obviously an ancient and creaky structure. It has endured for nearly twenty-four hundred years, sometimes as an inspiration, often as a museum piece. It has probably survived so long because it has never been given too much importance. It functions largely as a symbol of the ethical aspirations of the medical profession rather than as a regulatory document. There are many who would suggest that it is obsolete and should be abandoned. These arguments will be reviewed in detail in Chapter 2, but here we should note that the two major objections to the oath are that (1) it says little about the problems posed by modern technology and (2) its patient-centered orientation, now know as the "beneficence" principle, seems to foster an unwarranted paternalism on the part of the physician.

About the former criticism, I am suggesting that technology is not the problem that needs a solution, but rather the problem is a lack of a human or social context for applying that technology. The paternalism of modern medicine is much more a product of the Enlightenment ambition to control nature than of the ancient oath. What the oath has suggested throughout the centuries in its patient-centered strictures is the personalness of the relationship between the doctor and the patient, the importance of building and maintaining trust, and the importance of putting the needs and interests of the patient before those of the professional. How successful the medical profession has been in maintaining those ideals is a question worth asking. The codes should serve as professional beacons by which we check our course periodically.

Such checking may be difficult to do if the geography changes dramatically or if the siren song of commercialism appears too irresistible. However, if a radical change of course is required, it should not be made in a fog but with a sharp-eyed look at the alternatives.

8

Even though the Supreme Court has ruled that doctors have a "right" to advertise, this is not a right that was sought and is one that runs counter to the personal inclinations of most physicians. We have seen attempts of alternative providers to enter the marketplace, often those providing services in a personal manner not generally offered by the medical profession, but we have seen little overt professional advertising. There is competition in terms of different approaches to providing quality service, but these approaches are generally marketed by reputation, not advertising.

This model of professional restraint is one that widely prevails throughout the world, but one place where one can witness divergent approaches to the marketing of services is in Australia, where physicians have become split into two different camps. One group aggressively markets its services in a frankly commercial manner with advertising, price specials, and popular appeals. The other attempts to establish itself in the more traditional and perhaps slower manner of building trusted reputation in a community by providing quality service. This latter group identifies itself by the name "Hippocratic medicine."

I would suggest that the subtle but important human quality of trust in a personal professional-client relationship, which has characterized the Hippocratic tradition over the centuries, is especially crucial at a time of such uncertainty.[10]

PSYCHIATRY AND THE MEDICAL MODEL

Psychiatry as a profession rests on shaky grounds. It is part of medicine, but what does this mean for the identity of the psychiatrist? In considering psychiatry as a divided profession, we see that the division goes beyond the familiar divergences of treatment approach into more deep-seated epistemological divisions in our society.

Perhaps psychiatry could resolve its crisis of confidence by becoming closer to medicine. But if this is understood to mean limiting itself to the merely physical aspects of disease, then it risks buying into medicine's crisis of confidence. The so-called medical model has received a great deal of criticism for subjecting patients to a mechanistic process over which they have little control. This may be one of the reasons why informed consent, autonomy, and patient's rights have been receiving so much attention. But it is not at all clear that the medical model properly entails just a technological approach.

In its traditional sense, the medical model would be understood to involve the personal application of whatever techniques or remedies might be available to alleviate human suffering. It starts—as medical evaluation always has— with a personal assessment of the patient's needs: "Why have you come to me for help?"

Otto Guttentag, one of the first physicians to work in the philosophy of medicine, offers a useful definition of medicine that sets the medical model in its human context. "Medicine," he suggests, is "the care of health of human beings by human beings."[11] He distinguishes the "biological medical model" from the "anthropological medical model" as a reminder that there is more to medicine than the application of the laws of physics and chemistry.

The reminder should be especially useful for psychiatry, for the ethical dilemmas faced by psychiatry, like the ethical problems of the rest of medicine, cannot be understood, never mind solved, apart from an understanding of the social context in which they occur. What is right? What is good? What are the tensions we face as a society?

One tension is that between what can be precisely specified and what must remain ambiguous. Any practicing professional must cope with ambiguity in situations where precise certainty might be desired. Psychiatry is not unique in this regard. Furthermore, psychiatry is often called upon to resolve moral ambiguities, in the consulting room, in courtrooms, and in consultation to other branches of medicine. Thus it finds itself in tension with the legal system, with the rest of medicine, with other professions, and even with religion. These tensions may be taken as a source of confusion, but in fact they can be dynamic tensions, a source of creativity by which we can understand the relationship of the professions to the society in which they function.

This tension provides another reason for looking at ethics and psychiatry. Not only is the psychiatric profession brought into sharper focus by considering its ethical underpinnings, but also the nature of ethical conflict and reflection may be better appreciated by considering the contribution psychiatric thinking can make. Thus my tasks in this book are twofold: I attempt to show (1) that the conflicts that potentially divide the psychiatric profession may be reconciled by appreciating psychiatry's ethical basis as part of the medical profession, and (2) that the conflicts faced by the medical profession are conflicts that go deep to the heart of modern society, a fact that can be appreciated by considering the nature of the relationship between the professional and the person served.

George Engel, in arguing for a Bio-Psycho-Social Medical Model, has stated the problem nicely:

At a recent conference on psychiatric education, many psychiatrists seemed to be saying to medicine, "Please take us back and we will never again deviate from the 'medical model.'" For as one critical psychiatrist put it, "Psychiatry has become a hodgepodge of unscientific opinions, assorted philosophies and 'schools of thought,' mixed metaphors, role diffusion, propaganda, and politicking for 'mental health' and other esoteric goals." In contrast, the rest of medicine appears neat and tidy. It has a firm base in the biological sciences, enormous technologic resources at its command, and a record of astonishing achievement in elucidating mechanisms of disease and devising new treatments. It would seem that psychiatry would do well to emulate its sister medical disciplines by finally embracing once and for all the medical model of disease.

But I do not accept such a premise. Rather, I contend that all medicine is in crisis and, further, that medicine's crisis derives from the same basic fault as psychiatry's, namely, adherence to a model of disease no longer adequate for the scientific tasks and social responsibilities of either medicine or psychiatry. The importance of how physicians conceptualize disease derives from how such concepts determine what are considered the proper boundaries of professional responsibility and how they influence attitudes toward and behavior with patients. Psychiatry's crisis revolves around the question of whether the categories of human distress with which it is concerned are properly considered "disease" as currently conceptualized and whether exercise of the traditional authority of the physician is appropriate for their helping functions. Medicine's crisis stems from the logical inference that since "disease" is defined in terms of somatic parameters, physicians need not be concerned with psychological issues which lie outside medicine's responsibility and authority. At a recent Rockefeller Foundation seminar on the concept of health, one authority urged that medicine "concentrate on the 'real' diseases and not get lost in the psycho-sociological underbrush. The physician should not be saddled with problems that have arisen from the abdication of the theologian and the philosopher." Another participant called for a "disentanglement of the organic elements of human malfunction," arguing that medicine should deal with the former only.[12]

THE PROGRAM OF THIS TEXT

The chapters that follow are a series of essays that deal with the question of what defines a profession from a number of different, but related, points of view. They may be read separately, but taken as a whole they weave together the idea that a profession is defined by its ethics and specifically the ethic of human service.

Chapter 1, "The Place of Ethics in the Definition of a Profession," sets the stage by looking at the recent attempts of the Federal Trade Commission to redefine medicine as a trade rather than a profession. The ethics of professional advertising are the focal issue here. Professional advertising has long been held to be unethical by virtually every professional association in the world. But the FTC held that the AMA's code of ethics restrained trade because of the strictures against advertising and won the right to review any code of ethics that the AMA might promote. Here we see commercial considerations at the center of professional definition. It may be that medicine has become so business oriented that the FTC action is entirely credible. It certainly comes at a time of alarm about the growing costs of medicine (and medical technology) and enthusiasm for "market" solutions to problems of pricing. However, it also marks a clear departure from the traditional privacy of the doctor-patient relationship.

Chapter 2, "The Hippocratic Tradition in Medicine and Psychiatry," reviews the modern relevance of the Hippocratic Oath and related codes of ethics against the charge that they are obsolete. Here it is suggested that even now they maintain an important function by suggesting that the professional ethic is defined by the needs of those who come for help, not by the rival interests of society. Though constant tension always exists, this traditional notion continues to be important.

Appendices to Chapter 1 and Chapter 2 contain the text of the AMA's *Principles of Medical Ethics*, the Hippocratic Oath, and a "Hippocratic Oath for Psychiatrists" written by Maurice Levine.

Chapter 3, "The Tasks and Methods of Ethics," reviews some of the contributions of philosophy to ethical theories as well as some of the controversies about those theories. Ethics can be a system of rules, called the *deontological* approach to ethics, but they may also deal more broadly with the ends or goals of actions such as medical actions, called the *teleological* approach to ethics. Codes of ethics, while looking like a list of rules that function to enforce group standards of conduct, ultimately lack the specificity of deontological ethics and in fact function as principles to guide action. This ambiguity ultimately requires interpretation, which is one of the frustrations of ethics.

Chapter 4, "Confidentiality, Trust, and the Therapeutic Alliance," takes up one of the central themes of the Hippocratic tradition in ethics, namely, the importance of the privacy of the doctor-patient relationship, and illustrates some of the many threats to that privacy as society attempts to impose its own interests on the actions of the professional. The necessity of confidentiality for maintaining trust in a working partnership is suggested as an essential model not only for psychiatry but for all of medicine.

Chapter 5, "A Critique of Szasz's Critique: The Mind-Body Problem Won't Go Away," looks more closely at the ever-present tension between the mind and the body in modern medicine. Szasz bases his argument that mental illness is a myth on the simplistic idea that medicine should only deal with physical causes. This view is often implicitly held, but arguing it explicitly as Szasz does make the fallacy clear not only for psychiatry but for the larger problem of professional definition, where value judgments are inescapable in the problems that patients bring to their physicians.

Chapter 6 is titled "Informed Consent, Autonomy, and Paternalism: Respecting the Patient in Research and Practice." Informed consent has come to be a central tenet in modern medical ethics. It is seen as an antidote to the excesses of paternalism that accompany scientific medicine. The principle of autonomy, the right of the individual to self-determination, is seen by many as the basis for medical decision making. Autonomy is something that not everyone possesses, especially many psychiatric patients; thus something more fundamental is needed, the fiduciary doctor-patient partnership.

Chapter 7 is "The Place of Virtue and Character in Ethics: Psychiatry's

Contribution to Ethics." To be more than an impersonal analysis of alternatives, ethics must depend on the kind of people vested with decision-making authority; that is, professionals and their patients or clients. This chapter looks at the personal considerations involved in ethics, suggesting the contribution to ethics that psychiatry can make on a personal level. Psychiatry is concerned with the ancient admonition to know oneself. This approach to self-knowledge suggests avenues for teaching that go beyond abstract analysis of dilemmas or quandaries.

Chapter 8, "Idealism in Medical Ethics: The Pursuit of Moral Perfection," tries to sort out the difference between a moral imperative and a moral ideal. The development of a sense of self, a moral identity, through the mechanisms of the superego and ego ideal, is seen as a way of illuminating the workings of moral sensibility. It also points out the problems of confusing moral imperatives and moral ideals.

Chapter 9, "The Impeachment of Altruism," looks at the ideal of altruistic behavior for the medical profession and the tension with that ideal created by a self-interested society.

Chapter 10, "The Meaning of Medical Responsibility," looks at medical decision making not just as a balance between the interests of society and the interests of the individual or as a tension between the paternalistic authority of the physician and the autonomy of the patient. Rather, decision making is seen in terms of the response of the professional to the needs of those asking for help.

I hope to open these issues to a process of ethical reflection that will reaccredit the active, responsible, and responsive judgment of those who make decisions. One sees in the way I have juxtaposed these issues and questions a precarious oscillation between the political and the theoretical, which I would like to highlight at the outset as a roadmap of what is to follow. As we proceed down the paths opened to us by the considerations of medical practice and the reflections of ethics, I believe we will find these issues intertwined: the impersonal and grandiose ambitions of "man" to control nature, the scientific legacy of medicine; and the human desire to trust and be trusted, the humanistic legacy of medicine. Both these human inclinations are so deeply rooted in our philosophical traditions and so rigidly split in our minds that it is hard not to think of them as separate, mutually exclusive, and irreconcilable. Yet insofar as we are integral, whole human beings—persons of any moral integrity at all, not hopelessly fragmented—these dichotomous tensions are daily reconciled and integrated in all of us insofar as we do act responsibly under sometimes trying circumstances. I therefore take medical practice and the ethical reflection on that practice as an opportunity to review the philosophical traditions that shape the way in which we customarily view the world. At the same time I propose that a clarification of that worldview will help illuminate the problems that issue from medical practice.

13

CHAPTER 1

THE PLACE OF ETHICS IN THE
DEFINITION OF A PROFESSION

A SK ANY PERSON "What is a profession?" Medicine would certainly be mentioned. So would law. A profession is a way of earning a living, something one does, but not just any occupation. It involves higher education (the engineer? the scientist?) but also working with people and serving their needs. It is some higher calling, like the ministry or priesthood, perhaps the educator. Oh yes, doctors take the Hippocratic Oath, don't they? A profession requires commitment to ethical principles. You would want your children to belong to a profession when they grow up. But what is a professional? A basketball player? A violinist? Is it someone that helps you? A stock broker? An accountant? A military officer (once a legitimate vocation for the sons of the well-to-do)? Is it someone you can trust? A policeman? Is it someone with a high income and social prestige? A banker? What about "Yuppies," young urban professionals? They are well educated, ambitious, committed, affluent: doctors, lawyers, executives, entrepreneurs, movie makers, image makers.

If you asked a sociologist what characterizes a profession, you would probably get a much more specific answer. Sociological theory has looked closely at professions in terms of organization. Occupational groups from social workers to librarians to professional advertisers (marketers), following the model of physicians and lawyers, have developed university-based, specialized training programs, examinations, and professional organizations with a code of ethics, which can be used to include or exclude members of the professional group, a fraternity of like-minded individuals. The sociological view of a profession comments on the economic power of groups so organized—monopoly power is even mentioned—and the way professional organization is self-serving. It serves the economic interests of the professionals.

The sociological view of professions may sound jaded and cynical, especially to a professional who takes the ethical commitment seriously or even to the patient or client who is dependent on, has been helped by, and trusts his doctor or lawyer. But it must be acknowledged that the modern attitude toward professionals is ambivalent. Part of that ambivalence concerns the business or economic aspect of professional life. Part of it concerns the reliance on technique or knowledge in an abstract and seemingly uncaring

15

A PROFESSIONAL CHECKLIST [1]

1. The professional is engaged in a social service that is essential and unique.
2. The professional is one who has developed a high degree of knowledge.
3. The professional must develop the ability to apply the special body of knowledge that is unique to the profession.
4. The professional is part of a group that is autonomous and claims the right to regulate itself.
5. The professional recognizes and affirms a code of ethics.
6. The professional exhibits a strong self-discipline and accepts personal responsibility for actions and decisions.
7. The professional's primary concern and commitment is to communal interest rather than merely to the self.
8. The professional is more concerned with services rendered than with financial rewards.

---

way. However, there are two sides to ambivalence. The deeply felt appreciation for the professional stems from the ability to help someone in need. Yet even this is a source of ambivalence, for if there is anything that characterizes modern society, it is the desire to be independent and self-sufficient. The rejection of dependency is a virtue that becomes pathological in its extreme forms.

To consider oneself a professional places one in the middle of social tension. To be a professional means to place oneself in an attitude of service to one's fellow man, yet at the same time to earn one's living by the knowledge one has acquired. In this sense the professional and his or her patient/client are each dependent on the other. The relationship is symbiotic. To be a professional places one at the crossroads of an ethic of service and an ethic of economic opportunity. It would seem, gauging the pulse of modern sensibility, that the ethic of service is not as strongly felt as the ethic of economic opportunity. The sociological definition of a profession is convincing because it contains perceptible truth. But it is not the whole story. The ethic of service is inescapably part of what it means to be a professional.

THE DEFINITION OF A PROFESSION

The status of medicine as a profession has long gone unchallenged. If anything was a profession, it was medicine. Medicine, along with law and the clergy, the so-called "learned professions," were defined by the knowledge held by their members and by the application of that knowledge to the needs of fellow citizens. The relationship between the professional and those served was considered of special importance, and societies have traditionally placed

16

sanctions on that relationship, such as the protection of confidentiality, notable in English common law dating back to medieval times. But the sanctity of relationships with professionals has always existed alongside an uneasiness about the mercantile aspects of professional practice. Doctors especially often enjoy abundant remuneration along with the respect accompanying well-provided service. Chaucer commented on this when he noted that among the Canterbury pilgrims were a physician and an apothecary:

> They had known each other for a goodly while
> And each profited from the other's guile.

In the contemporary era, the criticisms of the medical profession have become so widespread that the idea of a profession being defined primarily by an ethic of service shared by its members is no longer entirely convincing. More prominent is the idea of a profession being defined by technical services traded in the marketplace. What does it mean for medicine to be considered a profession as distinct from a trade? Are the codes and traditions of ethics still relevant in defining medicine as a profession or will they have to be replaced by more explicit legal and regulatory definition?

Originally the word profession meant "to profess" religious vows. Medicine was a profession along with the clergy because its members shared a common "calling," and law was considered professional through a similar educational background in the medieval university.[2] University "professors" (the masters at the University of Paris) were first allowed to incorporate in the thirteenth century.[3] The debate about whether guilds and guild-like groups exert true monopoly power over prices has yet to be settled.[4]

What is considered professional might best be understood in contrast with what is not. In athletics as in sexual activity, the designation "professional" merely implies getting paid for what others do for free.[5] But the professional is also distinguished from the amateur by a greater level of proficiency that merits the monetary compensation. Thus some level of skill or expertise is generally held to be requisite for professional status. Reiser, Dyck, and Curran broaden this definition in a particularly useful way. They suggest that "Self-conscious reflection on standards of conduct is one of the defining characteristics of a profession."[6]

Thus professions are related to knowledge on the one hand and practice on the other. That places professions in an intermediate position between sciences and trades, with features in common with both but also features distinct from both.[7] The literature distinguishing professions from trades is abundant,[8-10] but in the twentieth century, as knowledge has come to mean scientific knowledge, the medical profession is increasingly identified with technical expertise. However, technical expertise is not sufficient to characterize a profession. The ethical dimension is also required.

THE SOCIOLOGY OF PROFESSIONS

A popular generalization in the sociological literature is that occupations are becoming "professionalized." Indeed courts and legislatures are witnessing challenges to professional territory as psychologists, nurse anesthetists, dental hygienists, and others lay claim to prerogatives that traditionally have been the exclusive domain of the medical and dental professions. But specialization, technical skills, and expertise do not suffice to establish a work group as a profession. What does? According to Wilensky, any occupation wishing to exercise professional authority must find a technical basis for it, assert an exclusive jurisdiction, link both skill and jurisdiction to standards of training, and convince the public that its services are uniquely trustworthy.[11]

The theme of trustworthiness is the pivotal criterion of professional status. The understanding of someone as a "professional" ultimately depends on the ability to trust that individual with personal matters. The various articulated codes of ethics of professional groups all stress the maintenance of the trustworthiness of members of the professional group through control of entry into and exit from the professional group and discipline of deviant members if necessary (for example, censure or removal from membership in the group, or removal of license). Table 1 illustrates the process of professionalization of a number of professions and would-be professions in the United States. It demonstrates that the route to professional status includes the establishment of university training programs, the formation of professional associations, and the presence of formal codes of ethics. The final step of public confidence is, of course, impossible to measure.

PROFESSION AND MONOPOLY

One of the most noticeable features of professional organizations, viewed in sociological perspective, is their attempt to control markets and promote self-interest. The theory of professional monopoly was developed by Max Weber, who described the following steps by which the medical profession, like all commercial classes, achieves monopoly power: creation of commodities, separation of the performance of services from the satisfaction of the client's interest (that is, doctors get paid whether or not the therapies work), creation of scarcity, monopolization of supply, restriction of group membership, elimination of external competition, price fixation above the theoretical competitive market value, unification of suppliers, elimination of internal competition, and development of group solidarity and cooperation.[12] Such careful delineation of an economic component to human motivation was truly radical in its time, but today it has become commonplace to reduce all human motivation to economic considerations.

The problem with this analysis of professional monopoly is that it is one-dimensional; it considers only economic motives and overlooks the

Table 1.

THE PROCESS OF PROFESSIONALIZATION*

	Became Full-time Occupation	First Training School	First University School	First Local Professional Association	First National Professional Association	First State License Law	Formal Code of Ethics
Established							
Accounting (CPA)	19th cent.	1881	1881	1882	1887	1896	1917
Architecture	18th cent.	1865	1868	1815	1857	1897	1909
Civil engineering	18th cent.	1819	1847	1848	1852	1908	ca. 1910
Dentistry	18th cent.	1840	1867	1844	1840	1868	1866
Law	17th cent.	1784	1817	1802	1878	1732	1908
Medicine	ca. 1700	1765	1779	1735	1847	Before 1780	1847
Others in process, some marginal							
Librarianship	1732	1887	1897	1885	1876	Before 1917	1938
Nursing	17 cent.	1861	1909	1885	1896	1903	1950
Optometry	1646	1892	1910	1896	1897	1901	ca. 1935
Pharmacy	17th cent.	1821	1868	1821	1852	1874	ca. 1850
School teaching		1823	1879	1794	1857	1781	1929
Social work	1898	1898	1904	1918	1874	1940	1948
Veterinary medicine	1803	1852	1879	1854	1863	1886	1866
New							
City management	1912	1921	1948	After 1914	1914	None	1924
City planning	19th cent.	1909	1909	1947	1917	1963	1948
Hospital administration	19th cent.	1926	1926		1933	1957	1939
Doubtful							
Advertising	1841	1900	1909	1894	1917	None	1924
Funeral direction	19th cent.	ca. 1870	1914	1864	1822	1894	1884

*Modified after Wilensky (*American Journal of Sociology* 70:137ff, 1964)

19

benefit to the public that occurs from such things as the promotion of scientific medicine and efforts to maintain professional standards.

The basic issue is whether physicians can place concern for the public good ahead of their own self-interest. Trust (or trustworthiness) is the keystone of medical virtue in the traditional canons of medical ethics from the Hippocratic Oath to Sir Thomas Percival's code—a nineteenth-century British code on which the first AMA code was based—to the various versions of the AMA codes. Trust is the basis of what it means to be a professional and what it means to be ethical. From the antitrust point of view, any trust, even basic human trust, is suspect as a form of monopolization. Berlant, applying Weber's theory of monopoly to the medical profession, states the case very cogently:

> [The] trust-inducing devices of the Percivalian code increase the market value of medical services and help convert them into commodities. . . . It also creates a paternalistic relationship toward the patient, which may undermine consumer organization for mutual self-protection, thereby maintaining consumer atomization. . . . Through atomization of the public into vulnerable patients, paternalism results in the profession's dealing with fragmented individuals rather than bargaining groups. Moreover, by appealing to patient salvation fantasies, trust inducement can stimulate interpatient competition by increasing each patient's desire to see that nothing stand between doctor and himself. Much of the emotional power of the sentiment of the doctor-patient relationship resides in this wish of the patient to save himself at any cost to himself or others.[13]

Berlant offers a sharp attack on professional ethics from a particular ideological perspective. But basically this attack is not just on professional ethics, but also on a kind of community in which people may not be autonomous and independent, but in which people may be dependent and in need of help that they willingly seek. This argument introduces a note of almost cynical suspiciousness into a society of individuals who seem almost too willing to trust and to place themselves in the care of others. This is a crisis of confidence— both for medicine and for our civic life in general: To what extent is it possible and necessary to trust and rely on others? To what extent is it possible to remain isolated, self-reliant, and autonomous human beings?

Table 2.

THE CODES OF ETHICS ON ADVERTISING

The Hippocratic Oath

Nowhere in the surviving Hippocratic writings do we find anything about advertising or self-promotion, but we do find a clearly established concept of the profession as a fraternity in the following statement: "I swear . . . to regard my teacher in this art as equal to my parents; to make him partner in my livelihood, and when he is in need of money to share mine with him; to consider his offspring equal to my brothers; to teach them this art, if they require to learn it, without fee or indenture; and to impart precept, oral instruction, and all the other learning, to my sons, to the sons of my teacher, and to pupils who have signed the indenture and sworn obedience to the physicians' Law, but to none other."

Percival's Code of Medical Ethics
Percival apparently had no occasion to refer explicitly to advertising on the part of English physicians, though his code is concerned throughout with maintaining the dignity, honor, and reputation of the profession.

AMA, 1847 Code
Duties of Physicians for the support of professional character: "It is derogatory to the dignity of the profession, to resort to public advertisements or private cards or handbills, inviting the attention of individuals affected with particular diseases—publicly offering advice and medicine to the poor gratis, or promising radical cures; or to publish cases and operations in the daily prints or suffer such publications to be made;—to invite laymen to be present at operations,—to boast of cures and remedies—to adduce certificates of skill and success, or to perform any other similar acts. These are the ordinary practices of empirics, and are highly reprehensible in a regular physician."

AMA, 1903 Revision
In this first revision after the Sherman Act, the caption "Principles of Medical Ethics" is substituted for "Code of Medical Ethics" leaving broader discretion to the state and territorial medical societies. The strictures against advertising specify methods to be avoided: "It is incompatible with honorable standing in the profession to resort to public advertisement or private cards inviting the attention of persons affected with particular diseases; to promise radical cures; to publish cases or operations in the daily prints, or to suffer such publication to be made; to invite laymen (other than relatives who may desire to be at hand) to be present at operations; to boast of cures and remedies; to adduce certificates of skill and success, or to employ any of the other methods of charlatans."

AMA, 1912 Revision
"Solicitation of patients by circulars or advertisements, or by personal communications or interviews, not warranted by personal relations, is unprofessional. It is equally unprofessional to procure patients by indirection through solicitors or agents of any kind, or by indirect advertisement, or by furnishing or inspiring newspaper or magazine comments concerning cases in which the physician has been or is concerned. All other like self-adulations defy the traditions and lower the tone of any profession and so are intolerable. The most worthy and effective advertisement possible, . . . is the establishment of a well-merited reputation for professional ability and fidelity. This cannot be forced, but must be the outcome of character and conduct."

AMA, 1957 Revision
A physician "shall not solicit patients." (A physician shall not attempt to obtain patients by deception.)

AMA, 1980 Revision
No comment on advertising in the *Principles of Medical Ethics,* as per FTC order. The *Current Opinions of the Judicial Council* (1982) offers the following comment:

21

"Competition between and among physicians and other health care practitioners on the basis of competitive factors such as quality of services, skill, experience, miscellaneous conveniences offered to patients, credit terms, fees charged, etc., is not only ethical but is encouraged."

British Medical Association, *Handbook of Medical Ethics* **(1981)**
"The medical profession in this country has long accepted the tradition that doctors should refrain from self-advertisement. In the Council's opinion advertising is not only incompatible with the principles which should govern relations between members of a profession but could be a source of danger to the public. A doctor successful at achieving publicity may not be the most appropriate doctor for a patient to consult. In extreme cases advertising may raise illusory hopes of a cure."

L'Ordre des Medecins, *Code de Deontologie Medicale (Belgium, 1975)*
Publicity, direct or indirect, is forbidden. The reputation of the physician is founded on his professional competence and on his integrity.

Canadian Medical Association, *Code of Ethics*
An ethical physician . . . will build a professional reputation based only on his ability and integrity, will avoid advertising in any form and make professional announcements according to local custom.

World Medical Association, *International Code of Medical Ethics*
Any self advertisement except such as is expressly authorized by the national code of medical ethics (is deemed unethical).

THE ANTITRUST CHALLENGE TO THE PROFESSIONS

A profession's service ideal has several manifestations: a formal code of ethics, more personal ethical outlooks, and certain activities—such as licensure, specialty certification, accreditation of institutions, and training programs—undertaken by a professional association to maintain standards of the group. It can be argued that such professional gatekeeping is an essential aspect of professional responsibility. However, a widespread perception exists that the restrictions that the learned professions have placed on themselves under the aegis of professional ethics have been motivated not in fact by "ethics" (in the sense of wanting to achieve a higher plane of moral conduct), but rather to serve the self-interest of the existing members of the profession.

Perhaps because of the ambiguous relationship of public interest and professional self-interest, the learned professions were considered exempt from the antitrust laws from the time of the passage of the Sherman Antitrust act in 1891 until the Supreme Court's *Goldfarb* decision in 1975, in which Virginia lawyers were found liable to charges of price fixing of the fees charged for title searches. The *Goldfarb* decision heralded a flurry of antitrust activity, most notably the suit by the Federal Trade Commission against the

American Medical Association, the Connecticut State Medical Society, and the New Haven County Medical Association, charging that these professional organizations were in restraint of trade because their code of ethics prohibited advertising. After a seven-year legal battle, this case was settled on March 23, 1982, when the Supreme Court split 4-4 leaving in place the lower court ruling that barred the AMA from making any prohibitive reference to advertising and the solicitation of patients in its code of ethics and further prohibiting the AMA from "formulating, adopting and disseminating" any ethical guidelines without first obtaining "permission from and approval of the guidelines by the Federal Trade Commission."[14] Though advertising is the focal issue in this particular case, the ethics of the profession both as explicitly formulated in the AMA's "Principles of Medical Ethics" and as implicitly practiced, as well as the right and propriety of a professional association to formulate its own code of ethics, are being called into question.[15, 16]

The FTC suit hinged on the questions of cost, advertising, and the mercantile aspects of the medical profession. The position of the FTC is that the reason costs are high is because doctors have a monopoly on health care delivery and can thus maintain artificially high costs for their own profit. If doctors were not prohibited from advertising, it is argued, prices would come down because patients could shop for the best deals. FTC chairman Michael B. Pertschuk stated the case as follows: "One possible way to control the seemingly uncontrollable health sector could be to treat it as a business and make it respond to the same marketplace influences as other American business and industries."[17] In other words, medicine could be better controlled if it were understood as a trade and not as a profession.

The categorization of medicine as a trade is obviously an oversimplification. The profession is inescapably concerned with the public well-being. Medicine is both a trade and a profession. It is certainly appropriate for the commercial aspects of medical practice to be regulated (or deregulated), but it would be a catastrophic mistake to assume that medicine is merely a trade and subject all aspects of professional regulation either to market influences or to the crude tools of antitrust litigation.

The courts have clearly recognized that professions have trade aspects. They have not eliminated the responsibility for professional self-regulation except in such instances in which such self-regulation may be in restraint of trade. For medicine the issue that the Supreme Court decided in *FTC v. AMA* is that the AMA's code of ethics cannot prohibit advertising. It remains for conscientious physicians to decide what constitutes ethical advertising.

THE ETHICS OF ADVERTISING

Medical advertising is at the crossroads of two very different philosophies about what medicine should be and how professions should be regulated. The traditional view opposes advertising to protect the public from physicians who are too commercially oriented. The more prevalent contemporary view holds that medicine is indeed commercially oriented and thus cannot be trusted to regulate itself. To reconcile the best aspects of traditional professionalism with the need for greater public accountability, it is necessary to consider what might be ethical and unethical in advertising.

Would advertising of physicians' fees and services be a desirable and ethical thing? If increased competition through advertising could reduce medical costs, then it would be socially desirable *unless* lowered costs were achieved through a lowering of the quality of service or *unless* increased advertising created a demand for more services, further straining the economy beyond the approximately 10 percent of the U.S. Gross National Product that currently goes to health care. The cost/quality equation is always a delicate balance. Although costs are easy to measure, the values by which we assess quality are impossible to quantify.

Advertising is a multifaceted issue. It serves two very distinct objectives: (1) the dissemination of information, and (2) product differentiation, which economists define as public perception of differences between two products, even though such differences may not in fact exist. The AMA has traditionally held that dissemination of information is acceptable, but that product differentiation or solicitation of patients is not.[18] The physician was to be distinguished from the itinerant merchant of nostrums by deemphasizing the commercial aspects of practice and emphasizing professional ethics (actually standards that minimized the differences that might exist between physicians similarly credentialed and certified). Thus if someone were to develop appendicitis while traveling in an unfamiliar part of the country, it would not be necessary to shop for a physician who believed in the germ theory or a hospital that maintained antiseptic standards. This shopping would be taken care of by credentialing procedures. The physician would obtain patients not by direct appeal to the public, but by building a reputation in a community. Although the distinction between dissemination of information and product differentiation was dropped in the 1980 revision of the AMA *"Principles of Medical Ethics,"* it remains an important distinction for physicians to keep in mind when contemplating the ethics of advertising. Advertising that provides information to consumers is ethical; creation of the illusion of differences through product differentiation is as unethical in medicine as it is in any business, even if not legally prohibited.

It could be debated whether advertising is ever ethical, though it is an accepted feature of capitalist societies. The ethical issue for advertising is whether advertising is truthful and whether there can be objectively measurable standards for judging the truthfulness of advertising claims. A more problematic concern is the way in which advertising plays upon people's unconscious wishes and fantasies: sex, greed, and the quest for power, status, and perfection. The scientific basis for advertising rests on the ability to identify and manipulate such longings and fears. When we speak of "the market" or "market forces" or "demand," we are generally talking about human wants and wishes.

Truthfulness in advertising was the concern when the field of advertising itself attempted to follow the course of professionalism in the early part of the twentieth century (see Table 1). At issue were the values that distinguished the professional advertisers from the retail-space merchants. The American Marketing Association (another AMA) established university training programs and codes of ethics that promoted the scientific ideal of detachment and statistical analysis. This scientific vision of community and definition of people (as consumers) replaced the older, empathic, and value-laden world in which a merchant had a feel for what his customers (not consumers) wanted because he lived with them in the same community.[19, 20] The transformation of medicine from an ethically based profession to a trade is nearly complete because it is commonplace to refer to the patient in the strictly commercial designation of "consumer."

The example of professional advertising is illustrative for the medical profession, not only because advertising promises (threatens?) to be such a conspicuous feature of contemporary medicine, but also because medicine's traditions of professionalism are derived from an era in which the physician participated in the life of the community in which he practiced. Knowledge of the patient as a person, as well as the patient's life history and social situation, has traditionally been deemed essential to quality care. At issue today for the profession of medicine is whether it will be possible to preserve the values of personal care that characterized the ideals of an earlier era. The ethics of medicine are derived from the time when medicine was a cottage industry. Will it be possible to maintain such ethics if medicine is transformed to assembly line efficiency?

CONCLUSION

It is paradoxical that medical ethics should be at the center of controversy about what is in the public interest. Ethical strictures against professional advertisement have a long and venerable tradition in the Western world, which stems from a view of professional life that cannot be easily reduced to economic analysis. The traditions represented by professional ethics stress the personal nature of professional practice. In the traditional model, trust is essential, for the patient/client must trust the professional to reveal such confidences as may be necessary to understand the problem. The professional is worthy of that trust according to (1) knowledge possessed and (2) such "professional" attributes as ability to keep confidences, to refrain from taking advantage of vulnerable patients, to put the patient's interests before one's own, and to refrain from self-aggrandizement at the patient's expense. It is out of such a view of professionalism that strictures against advertising arose.

The question of whether physicians should advertise cannot be settled until the prior question of what it means to be a profession is addressed. The economic analysis of market forces addresses a different concern from the concerns of professional ethics. The question is not whether doctors should be allowed to advertise, but what the trade-offs are with a strictly economic analysis of professional activities.

From the economic standpoint the question is this: Are there any reasons not to allow market forces to solve pricing and other problems? In other words, government regulation or professional self-regulation would be warranted only if the market fails. This is not the only question of interest, however. The ethical concern must also be addressed; namely, can quality care be maintained if the economically most efficient methods of health care delivery are adopted? From this point of view, the FTC strategy of reforming the medical profession by treating it as a business fails at the outset because it fails to consider the issues of quality care that are so much the concern of physicians and patients alike.

The message for the medical profession from the current round of antitrust litigation is clear: unfair trade practices will not be tolerated. A more subtle message must also be recognized: The reputation of the profession and its ethics have become tarnished as the public has come to perceive professional ethics as a protective mantle under which professionals cloak self-interest. This does not mean that the old ethics should be abandoned, but rather that they should be taken more seriously.

The doctor-patient relationship, spoken of almost religiously as the keystone of medical practice, has traditionally been a dyad in which the doctor answered directly only to the patient and his own conscience:

DOCTOR ◄──────────► PATIENT

In the modern era, financial considerations, even more than changes in technology, have transformed all parties in this relationship and added new ones:

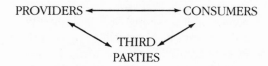

PROVIDERS ◄──────────► CONSUMERS

THIRD
PARTIES

Patients have become "consumers"; doctors have become "providers"; health care has become a commodity; and "third parties," including insurance companies, social service agencies, and allied health professionals, as well as corporate shareholders, are very much part of the picture. The patient seldom appears privately (and confidentially) to the doctor for help. Likewise the physician does not answer only to the patient. The conscientious physician concerned about cost containment may be put in the position of limiting the resources given to a demanding or anxious patient. Still the appeal of a person in need of help and the response of a concerned physician remain the essence of medical practice. Though some would suggest that medicine should, in the interests of efficiency, be limited to treating just physical ailments, most responsible physicians still concern themselves with the impact of disease and illness on people's lives and not just with the disease itself.

It is this broader concern of medical practice that professional ethics attempt to address and that is generally not understood to be an essential feature of a trade. The attempt to regulate the medical profession as a trade comes at a time when the activities of physicians are largely perceived as commercial and impersonal. Physicians must bear the responsibility for maintaining a broader concern for the patient as a person as part of their professional identity. To the extent that medicine fails in maintaining its professional ethical standards of public service and personal care, it is vulnerable to the criticism of self-serving commercialism. To the extent that medicine relies merely on technique and not on an ethic of service, it becomes merely a trade and not a profession.

APPENDIX 1

AMERICAN MEDICAL ASSOCIATION PRINCIPLES OF MEDICAL ETHICS

Preamble: The medical profession has long subscribed to a body of ethical statements developed primarily for the benefit of the patient. As a member of this profession, a physician must recognize responsibility not only to patients, but also to society, to other health professionals, and to self. The following Principles adopted by the American Medical Association are not laws, but standards of conduct which define the essentials of honorable behavior for the physician.

I. A physician shall be dedicated to providing competent medical service with compassion and respect for human dignity.

II. A physician shall deal honestly with patients and colleagues, and strive to expose those physicians deficient in character or competence, or who engage in fraud or deception.

III. A physician shall respect the law and also recognize a responsibility to seek changes in those requirements which are contrary to the best interests of the patient.

IV. A physician shall respect the right of patients, of colleagues, and of other health professionals, and shall safeguard patient confidences within the constraints of the law.

V. A physician shall continue to study, apply and advance scientific knowledge, make relevant information available to patients, colleagues, and the public, obtain consultation, and use the talents of other health professionals when indicated.

VI. A physician shall, in the provision of appropriate patient care, except in emergencies, be free to choose whom to serve, with whom to associate, and the environment in which to provide medical services.

VII. A physician shall recognize a responsibility to participate in activities contributing to an improved community.

ADOPTED JULY 22, 1980

CHAPTER 2

THE HIPPOCRATIC TRADITION IN MEDICINE AND PSYCHIATRY

THE MEDICAL PROFESSION is identified with the Hippocratic Oath. The Hippocratic Oath is symbolic of the ethical intentions and requirements of professional life for physicians. Patients and physicians alike—with only the vaguest notions of what the oath might actually entail—think of the oath as something morally binding on the physician and requiring obligations to the patient.

In recent years the Hippocratic Oath has been receiving renewed scrutiny. The headline ethical issues raised by new medical technology, increased costs, and changing social patterns have been the occasion for looking closely at whatever sources of wisdom might be useful in dealing with newly perceived problems. Under the harsh light of such critical scrutiny, the Hippocratic Oath has not fared well.

It is criticized, of course, for being outmoded and not dealing with the issues raised by the new medical technologies. It is also criticized for not dealing with the highest ethical principles that should govern the actions of physicians and for not articulating ethical principles according to the rights of patients. It is even criticized for arresting thinking about ethics.

The Hippocratic Oath's central tenet of the physician's obligation to the patient is also subject to criticism on the grounds that this attitude is paternalistic. All of these criticisms will be dealt with in turn, but it should be noted that all of these criticisms have a particularly "modern" cast. It should also be noted that we are on shaky ground if we judge historical tradition by the assumptions of a particular moment in history.

That the oath and the name of Hippocrates still remain in the popular mind as the highest symbol of the physician's dedication to healing and that the oath continues to encourage a fundamental bond of trust among the patient, the physician, and the medical profession suggest that close scrutiny is warranted not only of the Hippocratic writings but also of the tradition loosely based on them.

THE HIPPOCRATIC OATH

The Hippocratic Oath represents a small and largely ignored reform movement within the ranks of medical practitioners in the fifth and fourth centuries B.C. Its contemporary moral force was quite limited. The oath's prohibitions were morally binding only on proportionately few of those craftsmen who practiced ancient medicine. Most physicians in ancient Greece were not even aware of the oath's existence. Those that were chose to adopt or ignore whatever provisions of it they felt were relevant for them, based on their professional experiences, philosophical ideologies, and individual consciences.[1]

Historians tell us it was only around the tenth century A.D. under the influence of the Christian Church that the Hippocratic Oath came into widespread use. Most of the documents that survive are from this period. Early oaths, such as that ascribed to Hippocrates, were related to medical prayers. The supplication to the deities ("I swear by Apollo or whatever I hold most sacred"[2]) reflect the ancient practitioner's belief that success in his profession required that he ally himself with the deity in the treatment of disease. The supplication of the deities is intended to inspire the physicians to fulfill their moral obligations, reward those who honor their sacred trust, and punish those who violate it.[3]

The Hippocratic Oath was unique among the various ancient codes in its admonitions to make the healing of patients the single overriding feature of the physician's existence. The Hippocratic Oath proclaims a more strict morality for physicians than was established by Greek law, Platonic or Aristotelian ethics, or by common Greek medical practice. The physician was bound by the tenets applied to all citizens but also by special tenets that distinguished the physician from his fellow citizens.

By contrast an ancient Indian code, the *Charaka Samhita*, obliges the physician to deny services to enemies of his ruler, evildoers, unattended women, and those on the point of death. Thus the physician's obligations to the patient, though paramount, are subsumed to the interests of the "state."

Perhaps most important, the Hippocratic Oath represents the first time in the history of the world that the power to heal was vested in a practitioner who was not also a shaman with the power to harm. According to anthropologist Margaret Mead, the Hippocratic Oath marked one of the turning points in the history of man. Mead says, "For the first time in our tradition there was a complete separation between killing and curing. Throughout the primitive world the doctor and the sorcerer tended to be the same person. He with power to kill had power to cure, including especially the undoing of his own killing activities. He who had power to cure would necessarily also be able to kill."[4]

"With the Greeks," notes Mead, "the distinction was made clear. One profession, the followers of Aesculapius, were to be dedicated completely to life under all circumstances, regardless of rank, age, or intellect—the life of a slave, the life of the Emperor, the life of a child."

Mead observes that "this is a priceless possession which we cannot afford to tarnish," but society always is attempting to make the physician into a killer—to kill the defective child at birth, to leave the sleeping pills beside the bed of the cancer patient, and she is convinced that "it is the duty of society to protect the physician from such requests."

The pre-Hippocratic healers relied on exhortations of magic and supernatural powers. The modern physician, in what may come to be considered the post-Hippocratic era, is often relying on physiological interventions. The Hippocratic physician—from the earliest times with vestiges into the present —has relied on naturalistic observations, the rudiments of modern science, the powers of the body to heal itself in a proper environment with proper rest and nutrition, and the elusive but nonetheless important healing powers of caring individuals, family, friends, and the physician. Until quite recently the hope-giving power was probably one of the most important factors in the physician's healing skills. It would be hard to imagine that it does not remain important, though it may not be given due credence.

The naturalistic healing of the Hippocratic practitioner, of course, remains a vital concern for modern medicine. Despite several decades of preoccupation with the truly awesome advances in medical technology, there is a continuing and renewed awareness of the importance of a healthy lifestyle, proper nutrition, avoidance of noxious substances like tobacco, moderation in alcohol, and a stable social environment.

The Hippocratic Oath is also historically significant in that its strictures represent the first signs of professional organization. Those strictures are familial (actually fraternal) in nature and include the inclusion/exclusion feature and the regulation of conduct through a code of ethics, both of which have come to be associated with professional organization. The oath requires the apprentice physician to become essentially an adopted member of his teacher's family ("To hold him who has taught me as equal to my parents and to live my life in partnership with him"). It requires the student to help support his teacher and his teacher's children in case of need ("If he is in need of money to give him a share of mine, and to regard his offspring as equal to my brothers in male lineage"). Instruction is required to be passed on only to the teacher's children, one's own children, and to others who have sworn by the oath and thus in essence become members of the family ("To give a share of precepts and oral instruction and all the other learning to my sons and to the sons of him who has instructed me, and to pupils who have signed the, covenant and have taken an oath according to the medical law, but to no one else").

Thus by the establishment of family-like bonds between teacher and pupil, it was possible to maintain a careful selection of those admitted to the healer's group. The covenant enabled physicians to prevent persons judged unworthy from entering the profession.[5]

31

After establishing the nature of the contract between the teacher and student, the oath offers a number of specific injunctions, as described below.

Patient Confidentiality

Confidentiality has long been a central feature of the doctor-patient and of all professional-client relationships. The professional is bound to keep secret anything told to him in confidence; that is, in the course of the professional work. This confidentiality is essential if anyone is to trust a professional with important personal aspects of his life. Indeed the physician must rely on a recounting of the patient's history and be able to inquire of the patient about things the patient may not even have acknowledged to himself. This requires a high degree of trust.

The oath itself is more specific on the point of secrecy: "What I may see or hear in the course of the treatment or even outside of the treatment in regard to the life of men, which on no account one must spread abroad, I will keep to myself holding such things shameful to be spoken about." The aspects that we now consider as concerns for confidentiality were not so clearly formulated in Hippocratic times, but have come to be one of the essential features of professional life.

Abortion

The oath is quite explicit on the point of abortion. "I will not give to a woman an abortive remedy." This point of the oath is as controversial as is the question of abortion in modern society. Abortion was not generally considered unethical in Greek society, and the prohibition in the Hippocratic writings is another example of the stricter standards required of the Aesculapian fraternity.

Whatever the modern reader's views on abortion may be, it should be clear that abortion is not a simple matter, but represents a complex conflict of principles that goes beyond the simplifying rhetoric of rights—right to life, right to choice, right to caring parents. In its proscription against abortion, the oath stands against the trivialization of sex and pregnancy.

Euthanasia

The oath states, "I will neither give a deadly drug to anybody if asked for it, nor will I make a suggestion to this effect." This is difficult to interpret in light of the questions we now want to ask about definitions of death, turning off respirators, and quality of life. Even in the more simple Hippocratic times, it was clearly a proscription against the physician helping in the commission of suicide and, by extension, in what we would now consider mercy killing. It is the basis for the objection of the medical profession to a physician being used to give lethal injections in capital punishment. The proscription against "giving a deadly drug" implies a moral stand about such actions, but more important it defines the role of the physician as a unique participant in the affairs of society. The physician acts in the interest of the patient and refrains from being involved in interests that may conflict with those of the patient.

Truth-Telling

Though truth-telling is usually associated with the Hippocratic Oath, it is in fact probably a more recent virtue read back into the oath. The proscription in the oath usually associated with truth-telling has come to be associated with the injunction, "Whatever houses I may visit, I will come for the benefit of the sick, remaining free of all intentional injustice, of all mischief." Lying is a form of mischief. Thus the physician should carry out his treatment in a straight-forward, forthright manner.

However, there is always conflict as to what the truth entails and what is best for the patient. Elsewhere in the Hippocratic writings on etiquette (Decorum), the physician is urged not to reveal to patients "any gloomy assessment of their illnesses without careful forethought about the possible demoralizing effects it could have on them."[6] Thus within the Hippocratic writings as in so many situations in medicine, we observe a conflict of principles, to tell the truth but not to harm the patient. These conflicts are not resolved, indeed they cannot be resolved, without knowing the particular patient involved and thus relying on the judgment of the physician in a particular context. (The problems of truth-telling and lying will be considered further in Chapter 5.)

Sexual Contact with Patients

This is one of the forms of mischief that the Hippocratic code explicitly prohibits: "... remaining free of all mischief, and in particular of sexual relations with both female and male persons, be they free or slaves." This point is particularly relevant for psychiatrists and is the most *un*ambiguous point in the APA "Annotations Especially Applicable to Psychiatry" of the AMA "Principles of Medical Ethics": "Sex with a patient is unethical." Period. The reason for this prohibition in modern psychiatric terms is because of the awareness of the transferences that develop when a doctor is treating a patient and because of the dependency the patient may feel on the doctor. If the confidence is violated, the patient may have even greater difficulty forming trusting relationships.

Though this is the modern formulation, we notice the same concerns for the development of trusting relationships even in Hippocratic times. The proscription against "mischief" may be seen as an aspect of the trust-building aspects of the medical profession, relying on the formation of trusting rela-tionships as one of the healing powers of the physician. We notice also that the physician refrains from taking advantage of opportunities that might be uniquely available to him, thus distinguishing himself in society by virtue of ethical standards that not everyone would be expected to adhere to.

The prohibition about sex with patients (and of course former patients since transferences endure in time) is of crucial importance for psychiatrists. But the issues of trust and dependency are no less relevant for other physicians.

Professional Affiliations

The Hippocratic Oath introduces the idea that the physician restricts his area of practice and affiliates with those who adhere to similar values. ("I will not use the knife, not even of sufferers from the stone, but will withdraw in favor of such men as are engaged in this work.") Though this part of the code is now anachronistic, we see in it the shaping of the modern medical profession. Surgeons have now been incorporated into the fold as surgical techniques have improved, though in Great Britain, surgeons are still referred to as "Mister" rather than "Doctor." Nonetheless the prohibitions against associating with "non-scientific practitioners" that are found in various versions of both the British and American medical codes have their origin in the Hippocratic Oath.

Justice in the Distribution of Health Services

The oath requires the physician to "remain free of all intentional injustice." The Greek term *adikie*, which is translated as "injustice," has the broader meaning of "wrongdoing" and thus its inclusion alongside "mischief." Today we usually understand this requirement as a duty to deliver health care equitably. This concept—of equal treatment for males and females, free and slave—was novel in Hippocratic times, as expressed by the suggestion to refrain from sex equally with men or women, free or slave.

Patient Benefit

Taken as a whole, the central tenet of the Hippocratic Oath and tradition is the benefit of the patient. The physician must subsume self-interest to what is good for the patient. This patient-benefit principle is often tagged with the epithet, *Primum Non Nocere*, "First Do No Harm," though this is not in fact from the Hippocratic Oath itself, but found elsewhere in the Hippocratic corpus.

THE CASE AGAINST HIPPOCRATIC MEDICINE

It is clear that the Hippocratic writings emerged from a time and a culture very different from our own . What is striking is that the Hippocratic tradition has endured so long, its twenty-four hundred year legacy making it one of history's most enduring institutions. We can witness in the Hippocratic writings the shape of the contemporary medical profession as we know it today.

Tradition is not virtue in itself, of course. And the objections to the Hippocratic Oath hinge on the same kind of debates as one hears about the relevance of history. On the one hand, those that don't heed the lessons of

THE HIPPOCRATIC TRADITION

history are doomed to repeat the mistakes of the past. On the other, a preoccupation with history impedes progress.

It is useful to take up the objections to the Hippocratic tradition in sequence:

The Hippocratic Oath is anachronistic

This argument relies on the perception of contemporary medicine as largely technological. There is little in Hippocratic times that could anticipate the dilemmas posed by advanced life-support systems, interchangeable parts, experimental drug therapies, diagnosis by imaging and chemical analysis, and newer reproductive technologies like in vitro fertilization.

It is often argued that such technologies have reshaped the goals of medicine and rendered the Hippocratic outlook obsolete. Since the Hippocratic Oath came into being in primitive times vastly different from our own, it cannot be expected to offer much guidance in contemporary problem solving. The sooner we recognize this the better. Altman suggests that "The Hippocratic Oath is a museum piece, an amiable but useless custom."[7]

The Hippocratic Oath doesn't deal with the highest ethical obligations of the physician

This objection appears in various forms. Carlton Chapman, for example, observes that

> For centuries the Oath has been viewed sentimentally and uncritically by the medical profession as its ethical standard and has, rather paradoxically, served as a barrier to the development of an adequate and comprehensible ethical statement for the profession.[8]

Basically the code falls short for not adequately stressing the "rights" of patients or for stressing too much the relationships of physicians to each other.

Chauncey Leake voiced a similar objection to Percival's code of ethics, an eighteenth-century descendant of the Hippocratic code and predecessor of the AMA codes, on the grounds that what it was dealing with were matters of etiquette, not ethics.[9]

The Hippocratic Oath opposes abortion and euthanasia

Some object to the strictures against abortion and voluntary euthanasia embodied in the Hippocratic Oath since they are phrased in absolute terms, admitting no exceptions whatever. These two prohibitions, along with restrictions against infanticide and suicide that the Oath tacitly implies, need to be loosened or abandoned, critics allege, in view of biomedical developments like amniocentesis and heart-lung machines, which have greatly expanded our options.

Hippocratic medicine has been faulted for defining medical care mainly in terms of emergency treatment

The oath says little about preventive and ongoing approaches to medical treatment. However, in the Aesculapian treatments on the island of Cos, a spa-like emphasis on rest, nutrition, and healthful living was an important aspect of health care.

The patient benefit principle of the Hippocratic writings is paternalistic

We have seen that the Hippocratic conception of the physician-group was that of a family organization. Similarly the physician's attitude toward the sick patient is analogous to the concern of a parent for a child. Throughout history this paternalism has been the hallmark of medical virtue. What higher testimony could there be to the physician's dedication than to say that he cared for his patients with the same devotion as he would his own children?

In recent years social attitudes have begun to change. While some people still "put themselves in the hands of physicians," others are finding paternalism objectionable. The requirement that the physician act for the benefit of the patient requires the physician to make a judgment as to what is best for the patient. This sometimes manifests itself as a "Doctor Knows Best" attitude, which might understandably be objectionable. Indeed the physician's judgment of what is best for the patient and the patient's judgment might come into conflict, as for example in how much to tell a patient about what is going on. Though judgment can be fallible, the emphasis on patient benefit in the Hippocratic Oath conceivably encourages the physician to make judgments on behalf of patients, judgments that patients might appropriately make for themselves.

The philosopher Robert Veatch most strenuously objects to this aspect of the Hippocratic tradition, and he does so on grounds of patient autonomy. The autonomous patient can and should be making decisions for himself and would not want to make himself dependent on a physician or to substitute the physician's judgment for his own.[11]

IN DEFENSE OF THE HIPPOCRATIC TRADITION

It seems that one of the most damning criticisms that has been leveled against the Hippocratic Oath is that it is not modern. Unless we are prepared to accept the contemporary outlook as the reference standard for values, we must look more critically not only at the oath, but also at the criticisms of the oath.

First of all we must ask, "Is modern medicine synonymous with high technology?" High technology is clearly a part of modern medicine, but is it an end in itself? If we do not accept medicine as identical with high technology, then the criticism that the Hippocratic code does not offer guidance for dealing with technology becomes less important. Indeed the oath may well

offer guidance for dealing with technology in the suggestion that the technological tools we now have available are subservient to the human goals of
medicine.

The second objection to the Hippocratic Oath presents us with a similar
dilemma. Does the Hippocratic Oath fail us in articulating the highest ethical
principles that should govern the conduct of physicians? Clearly it says little
about the rights of patients to which we now give so much accord. It focuses
on the obligations of the physician. However, the concept of patient's rights is
also subject to problems, notably the isolationist and self-centered outlook of
the autonomous position. These problems will be considered further in the
chapter on informed consent (Chapter 6). Here it is sufficient to note that the
concerns of the Hippocratic Oath with the relationship of the physician to the
patient may be more relevant than recent philosophical trends would at first
want to acknowledge.

Similarly the emphasis on "etiquette" in the Hippocratic Oath and its
latter day derivatives may also have its place in establishing a sense of
community and predictability among practitioners. Such etiquette may have a
legitimacy both in providing guidelines to practitioners and in helping patients know what to expect.

The third objection to the code that we need to consider is that the
prohibitions against abortion and euthanasia are phrased as absolutes, admitting no exception. About this objection I think there are two considerations.
First of all, it is a mistake to read the oath too closely as a list of rules. Rather it
makes more sense to understand it symbolically in terms of the intent and the
concept of the profession it outlines. Even so, the prohibitions against abortion and euthanasia have a relevance that may still be worth considering. The
situations in which abortion might be morally considered are not necessarily
done so without tragic considerations. That is, one does not need to say that
abortion is a good thing to recognize that situations exist where the absence
of a choice would be worse. The guarantee by the U.S. Supreme Court in 1973
in *Roe v Wade* of a "right" to abortion (under certain circumstances) deals
with a different sort of question than the moral "good" of a particular decision.
Thus it is most appropriate that the idea of an ethical standard be preserved,
apart from the legal considerations of what the state may require or prohibit.
The presence of the Hippocratic Oath serves as just such a reminder.

The same may be said about euthanasia. The presence of heart-lung
machines and artificial ventilators has really done little to change the meaning
of death or dying. They have forced a rethinking of the physiological processes in the event of dying. But the goal of the physician in preserving life is
altered not at all by the presence of life-extending technologies.

The question that does arise has to do with the application of such
technologies to the goals of medicine. It is often asked, "Why, if one is going to
let a person die, does one not kill that person instead? Would that not be more
humane, more logically consistent?" Though the logical coherence of such

arguments is usually recognized, the physician almost invariably sees the goal of medicine to preserve life, rather than take life, so much so that life is often equated in a reductionistic way with cellular metabolism. Thus the physician may fail to stop the senseless application of technology, which of course is hardly required.

The objection to paternalism in the Hippocratic tradition warrants the most serious consideration because it represents one of the most sensitive points in contemporary society. Any physician is familiar with the patient who in time of need trustingly defers to medical judgment. Yet also familiar is the patient who questions every recommendation, reads about medications and treatment, and inquires about the latest research reports. Indeed the informed patient makes a good partner in health care.

The issue of paternalism in the Hippocratic tradition is not necessarily at odds with the modern goal of autonomy unless one conceives of medical decision-making as more or less an instantaneous act. Unfortunately, this may often be the case in the modern medical setting. The relationship between doctor and patient may hardly be more enduring than that between a shopkeeper and customer.

For all its lack of favor among some, paternalism is not, strictly speaking, opposed to autonomy, as is so often argued. The responsibilities of the wise parent toward the dependent child are to promote growth and autonomy. Similarly, such attitudes are still appropriate for physicians toward patients, who at times of sickness may need to be dependent but whose autonomy should be encouraged as they assume more control over and responsibility for many aspects of their own health care and health promotion. This view of medical care is a relationship that endures over time.

Perhaps no aspect of the Hippocratic code is more significant than the focus on the interests of the individual patient. So familiar has this aspect of Western medicine been for so long that it is sometimes difficult to imagine what medicine would be like if the interests of the patient were not held foremost. The physician in the Hippocratic tradition functions as an agent of the patient. But there are many places and many situations in which the physician may be asked to serve other interests, such as interests of the state.

CONFLICTING DEMANDS UPON THE PHYSICIAN

The alternative to the Hippocratic tradition can best be appreciated by listing some of the demands that may be placed on physicians. Such a listing suggests the importance of the physician being bound by a unique professional ethic, which is neither one that applies to all people equally nor one that admits to any compromise with the "common good." The following are some of the situations in which interests other than the benefit of the patient may be brought to bear on the physician:

Cooperation with torture

The Nuremberg trials brought to light numerous examples of physicians cooperating with the Nazi government during World War II. This occasioned a more explicit codification in the Geneva Principles of earlier Hippocratic principles. Recently we have become aware of examples of physicians cooperating with military governments, particularly in Latin America, in the torture of political prisoners. Such torture is often justified as "in the interest of the state," even though it is of course in violation of human rights as well as the Hippocratic tradition. The role of the physician may vary from sadistic enjoyment in the application of the torture to the more common pattern of assisting, perhaps under threats and other coercion, in examining the prisoner to see if he can tolerate more torture.

Professional societies, such as those I had an opportunity to visit in Brazil, have acted against such physicians in much the manner of many professional societies that attempt to discipline members who do not adhere to their codes of ethics. In Brazil, like many of the continental European countries (but unlike the Anglo-American tradition), the codes of ethics of the professional organizations have the standing of law. This is often argued as desirable by those who say the state should be more involved in the regulation of the professions. However, when physicians act in the interest of the state, this involvement can have undesired effects. In Brazil the sanctions imposed by the medical society were overturned by the government, which has the ultimate authority because the accused physicians were working for the government. What an autonomous professional body might lack in terms of the "teeth" of a governmental agency, it stands to gain in terms of moral independence through allegiance to a higher ethic.

Political abuse of psychiatry

A more subtle but no less disturbing abuse of the medical profession occurs in several Eastern European countries, notably the Soviet Union, in which political dissidents are detained in psychiatric hospitals, allegedly suffering from "mental disturbances." Again the physicians involved may be subject to varying degrees of subtle and not-so-subtle forms of coercion, creating dilemmas at the level of individual conscience. However, the moral outrage of the international community, as voiced by the World Psychiatric Association in the code of ethics drafted in the late 1970s to respond to this phenomenon, helps provide physicians with an ethical "touchstone" independent of state judgment.

Lethal injections in capital punishment

The American Medical Association has gone on record as opposing the participation of physicians in capital punishment. The physician's ethic with its Hippocratic derivatives requires the physician to aid the patient and not be an agent in killing. This is not quite the same thing as opposing capital punishment, which is not an issue that comes under the physician's concern for an individual patient, though it is certainly an issue that individual physicians may have strong convictions about, just as they may have strong convictions about gun control or nuclear disarmament. Although lethal injections may be more "humane" than other forms of capital punishment, it is not the place of the physician to participate in such actions.

Cost containment

There has been increasing awareness for at least the past two decades of the need for physicians to help contain high medical costs. This imperative could create a conflict of interest if the physician assumes the responsibility of acting as society's agent in limiting the amount of care an individual patient may receive. The Hippocratic Oath serves as a point of reference in resolving the tension between the conflicting obligations a physician may feel in mediating the interests of individuals and the larger interests of society.

SUMMARY

The oath and the name of Hippocrates still remain in the popular mind the highest symbols of the physician's dedication to healing. The oath continues to encourage a fundamental bond of trust among the patient, the physician, and the medical profession, and it promotes a concern for the individual patient that goes beyond other interests that may impress themselves upon the physician.

Though at first glance the oath may appear outmoded on several counts, it still remains surprisingly relevant to contemporary medical ethical concerns.

Carrick suggests that there are two reasons for the oath's relevance:

> First, it continues to center the attention of society on a basic core of perennial medical ethical issues that constitute virtually ineliminable categories of legitimate moral concern that we ignore only at our own peril.
>
> Second, it affirms the importance of the graduate physician's covenant (or public promise) to be professionally committed to and so morally responsible for: (a) the physical and psychological welfare of patients who trustingly, and often naively, seek medical relief from their assorted maladies; and (b) the technical competence and moral integrity of himself as well as his or her medically trained peers.[12]

Ultimately the most strenuous criticism of the Hippocratic Oath may prove to be its greatest strength. It is not modern. Judged by the standards of the present, the oath fails to offer specific guidelines on a number of important points. But as a reference for judging the standards of the present, the oath offers a very useful perspective. It gives us a perspective on ourselves so that we do not take our beliefs for granted, and it prevents us from sanctifying the whims of the present.

Appendix 1

OATH OF HIPPOCRATES[13]

I swear by Apollo Physician and Asclepius and Hygieia and Panaceia and all the gods and goddesses, making them my witnesses, that I will fulfill according to my ability and judgment this oath and this covenant:

To hold him who has taught me this art as equal to my parents and to live my life in partnership with him, and if he is in need of money to give him a share of mine, and to regard his offspring as equal to my brothers in male lineage and to teach them this art—if they desire to learn it—without fee and covenant; to give a share of precepts and oral instruction and all the other learning to my sons and to the sons of him who has instructed me and to pupils who have signed the covenant and have taken an oath according to the medical law, but to no one else.

I will apply dietetic measure for the benefit of the sick according to my ability and judgment; I will keep them from harm and injustice.

I will neither give a deadly drug to anybody if asked for it, nor will I make a suggestion to this effect. Similarly I will not give to a woman an abortive remedy. In purity and holiness I will guard my life and my art.

I will not use the knife, not even of sufferers from the stone, but will withdraw in favor of such men as are engaged in this work.

Whatever houses I may visit, I will come for the benefit of the sick, remaining free of all intentional injustice, of all mischief and in particular of sexual relations with both female and male persons, be they free or slaves.

What I may see or hear in the course of the treatment or even outside of the treatment in regard to the life of men, which on no account one must spread abroad, I will keep to myself holding such things shameful to be spoken about.

If I fulfill this oath and do not violate it, may it be granted to me to enjoy life and art, being honored with fame among all men for all time to come; if I transgress it and swear falsely, may the opposite of all this be my lot.

Appendix 2

HIPPOCRATIC OATH FOR PSYCHIATRISTS

What follows is an oath in the Hippocratic tradition drafted for psychiatrists. It was written by Maurice Levine, distinguished former chairman of the University of Cincinnati Department of Psychiatry, and published in his book *Psychiatry & Ethics*.[14] Levine demands competence, but recognizes that human beings are not perfect. His code articulates the very important principle about the importance of self-knowledge or at least self-awareness and constant self-scrutiny, which is a venerable notion in ethical traditions, but which goes beyond the requirements of the American Psychiatric Association's (APA's) *Annotations Applicable to Psychiatry*. Though Levine's ideas are in no way officially binding on psychiatrists, they well deserve to be kept in mind, for they offer guidance in problems that have brought many psychiatrists before the APA Ethics Committee on complaints of unethical conduct from their patients. His suggestion of the importance of consultation and particularly the kind of consultation called supervision bears careful consideration. The emphasis on the cooperative team effort as a form of trusting alliance is an important cornerstone of professional ethics.

HIPPOCRATIC OATH FOR PSYCHIATRISTS

I am deeply moved by the fact that my profession is one which has high human ideals and aspirations. I know that psychiatrists are not perfect and need not be, but I profoundly honor their attempt to do a good job and to practice their profession with honesty and self-respect. I know that I too am far from perfect, but I will make a sincere attempt to do a really decent job. I shall certainly follow the good advice of the Hippocratic Oath. I shall avoid the felonies, the misdemeanors, and the misbehavior referred to in the original oath. And if ever I find myself doing a medical treatment for which I am not prepared, or trying to be seductive to a patient, I will recognize that I have a serious neurotic disorder, and try to get treatment. If I am unable to bring myself to treatment, I will give up my work with patients or confine my activities to fields in which there will be no temptation.

And even though I have no such obvious neurotic reactions to my patients, I often will turn my eyes and ears inward, to see if in any way my own emotional attitudes are keeping me from functioning at my best level. I know that patients will respond inappropriately far more often than I will, but I will not hide behind that fact. Indeed, each physician of any specialty or in general practice must be aware of his own attitudes and thoughts and feelings, to see if at any time they are interfering with the quality of his work with patients. As a psychiatrist, I have that obligation even more than do other physicians. And no matter what treatment I use, I will examine my choice with care. I will not give

42

drugs because I am impatient, nor use psychotherapy because I have free time.

I will observe myself as well as my patients. And if, in this recurrent process of stringent self-scrutiny, at any time I detect in myself too much anxiety, too much sympathy, too much coolness, or too much conceit, or diffidence, or leniency, or strictness, or any other excessive attitudes, I will make an honest attempt to modify them by my own efforts.

But I shall not permit such a stringent honesty to become a new kind of scrupulosity, a new kind of hairshirt, or a striving for superhuman perfection. I know that training in medicine, and training in psychiatry, these days is good enough so that the relationship of most psychiatrists with most patients, even in the more subtle issues, is very workable indeed. But if an inappropriate attitude or response to a patient persists in spite of my efforts, I will arrange at my own expense for a period of the kind of consultation which is called supervision, in which another experienced psychiatrist will consider thoroughly my work with the patient. And fortunately such an expense is tax-deductible!

Further, in such supervision I will avoid breaking confidentiality. I will change the identifying facts about the patient so as to conceal his identity and the identity of anyone mentioned by him.

If, however, even after a stringent self-scrutiny, I do not see any issues in my own personality that interfere with my work, I shall breathe a sigh of relief.

But, if my self-scrutiny does not convince me definitely one way or the other, but, as a third possibility, leaves me uncertain and uncomfortable, I shall consider the various ways of having a check by others on my work. Under these circumstances, I could arrange for some hours of supervision, of the sort mentioned above. Or, I could discuss my work, preserving confidentiality, with a contemporary, who I know will not withhold criticism and suggestions out of his friendship with me.

Or, if I work in a group or in a hospital or in a clinic in which there are active staff discussions of patients in treatment, I shall arrange to present my case—material for critical discussion and suggestions—again preserving confidentiality.

And I shall give serious consideration to a plan which may be the best of the alternatives. This would be to join, or to organize, a small seminar group of peers, to present and to discuss the work of each in rotation. Such a seminar might consist of three to five psychiatrists, meeting at regular intervals, in an arrangement which could continue for many years after my training is over. The psychiatrists of such a group would be chosen on the basis of competence and congeniality and friendship, so that each can feel that the comments of the others are essentially helpful even when they are critical.

In such a seminar, I will present samples of my work for evaluation, hoping that the others will comment on the strong points of my work which I then can develop further, and hoping further that they will notice any mistakes which I had not noticed, and make productive suggestions for a change. Such a group could play a vital role in my continuing development.

Before joining such a seminar, I will take an oath far more difficult than any portion of the Oath as written by Hippocrates. I promise to present to the group not only examples of work which I think were good, but also examples of work about which I was doubtful, and especially examples of my work taken at random. And in such a seminar as in the other plans, I will preserve confidentiality.

And I hope very deeply that I will retain perspective about myself, that I never will think that being a psychiatrist means living on Mount Olympus. Rather I will use images about myself that are far from godlike. I will merely hope that in my work I can improve my batting average, that I can stay on the fairway, and that the patient and I can form a cooperative team to work toward his improvement and cure.

For I know that it is not necessary to feel that I am Olympian, nor to feel small and helpless. I know that it is enough to belong to the human species, to be at the level of men and women, strengthened by thorough training. Then the practice of psychiatry can be infinitely rewarding in the satisfactions of human helpfulness.

We, as psychiatrists, will not give up when we stumble. Our job has rough moments, but it is enormously worth doing, it is idealistic but practical, and it is thoroughly alive. We hope deeply that we can grow in stature as we practice, not only in our scientific and technical knowledge and ability, but also in our strength, our maturity, and our integrity. This is our hope, our Oath.

CHAPTER 3

THE TASKS AND
METHODS OF ETHICS

IN A HOMOGENEOUS culture, tribe, or community, morality is tacitly understood with little need for formal reflection or articulation. One learns the rules of culture by living in that culture and not by being taught abstract and explicitly formulated rules. In a heterogeneous group, what we call a "pluralistic society," there may be little adhesion to shared principles.

In a stable culture, moral norms are internalized, and we think of ethics as matters of conscience. In a changing culture, the internalized morality of a particular subgroup or individual may be in conflict with other mores, and we may not trust that the dictates of individual conscience are an adequate safeguard of right conduct. Increasingly in this society we are moving away from informal standards of both personal and professional ethics, from broad and tacitly indwelt general principles developed over centuries, toward a civilly enforced body of laws and administrative regulations. This change has been interpreted as resulting from a deep current mistrust of all "assumed relationships"; that is, the breakdown of *Gemeinschaft* (a community of feeling that results from likeness and shared life experience) into *Gesellschaft* (a more rational, more mechanistic way of life, with greater structure and more written and explicit rules and regulations.)[1] Broad ethical principles no longer serve as shared values, and there is an attempt to make moral principles explicit as behavioral guidelines.

WHAT IS ETHICS? MEDICAL ETHICS?

What then is ethics? It is more than morality, the values of a particular culture. In fact ethics may be said to result from the process of reflecting on a given set of values, particularly as they are translated into action, often in a preconscious, prearticulate fashion. A working definition of ethics varies considerably depending on one's perspective, which should be no surprise.* Medical

---

*The terms *ethics* and *morals* are often used interchangeably. Most of the new breed known as ethicists agree that ethics (singular) or medical ethics is a discipline, a science, or a method of

ethics are related to but not limited to the norms of medical practice. Medical ethics also reflect the values of the culture in which medicine is practiced. Chauncey Leake, a pharmacologist and early commentator on medical ethics, notes that what is usually referred to as medical ethics is really more a matter of professional etiquette. He writes in the preface to his edition of *Percival's Medical Ethics*, which served as exemplar for the early AMA codes:

> The term "medical ethics" introduced by Percival is a misnomer. Based on Greek traditions of good taste . . . it refers chiefly to the rules of etiquette developed in the profession to regulate the professional contacts of its members with each other. . . . Medical etiquette is concerned with the conduct of physicians toward each other and embodies the tenets of professional courtesy. Medical ethics should be concerned with the ultimate consequences of the conduct of physicians toward their individual patients, and toward society as a whole, and it should include consideration of the will and motive behind this conduct.[2]

Dan Clouser, a philosopher teaching in a medical center, notes that "Medical morality is no different than normal, everyday morality. . . . It is just that in medical ethics these familiar moral rules are being applied to situations and relationships."[3] Charles Moore, a practicing physician who spent a year at the Hastings Center studying medical ethics, wrote his reflections of his experiences there in an article entitled, *"This* is medical ethics?" He noted that, "Most of the conversations I have had with ethicists have tended to anger me, producing a feeling of deep frustration." He identified the reason for this frustration as the fact that most ethicists dealt with research issues and not with the issues facing the practicing physician.[4] I suspect there may have been deeper reasons as well, such as the gulf between the respective worlds of discourse of the physician and the ethicists. At the very least these vignettes suggest that there is considerable difference of opinion as to what medical ethics are or should be.

What the word "ethics" connotes may be very different to a physician, reflecting on daily practice, and a philosopher, criticizing those practices from without. What I am suggesting is not just a mutual antagonism, though that may be an ingredient, but a difference of perspective, a difference involving the distinction of self and other. Both approaches are legitimate and relevant. Yet confusion often arises when one speaks about "ethics" as to whether one intends to be self-reflective or critical. If one adopts a self-reflective stance, one opens oneself to the scrutiny of others. If one takes a critical stance, one runs the risk of making others defensive. Ethicists are commonly perceived as critics of the moral behavior of others, even sometimes as scolds; therefore, it is important to keep sharply in focus the nature of the ethical enterprise one is undertaking.

reflection. This usage goes back to Aristotle, whose "Nicomachean Ethics" is still a standard point of reference. Ethics (noun, plural) refers to the norms of a group and in this usage may mean the same thing as morals (e.g., "their ethics [or morals] are questionable").

The ethical orientation of the modern practitioner of medicine is particularly problematic. The contemporary physician is caught between the *Gemeinschaft* of traditional medical ideals and the *Gesellschaft* of regulatory guidelines. Traditions at least as old as the cults of Aesculapius and the Oath of Hippocrates stress the fiduciary character of medical practice: The fundamental warrant of medical practice is the trust placed in the physician, based on the physician's competence and intention to help or benefit the patient. But being traditional, these ideals are largely unarticulated and inherently ambiguous. In recent years ever more explicit codification has supplemented the received traditions.[5]

An important distinction for medical ethics hinges on the notion of a profession. It has been suggested that self-conscious reflection on standards of conduct is one of the defining characteristics of a profession.[6] Ethical reflection for a profession consists of setting standards, often articulated as ethical codes, then judging its members for inclusion or exclusion by those standards. Here the concern is as much with the moral reputation of the professionals as a group as with the moral integrity of a particular member.[7]

Often there is no explicit statement as to the expected behavior of the professional, but through "socialization" or "professionalization" the physician comes nonetheless to understand what is expected. I often ask medical colleagues from other countries how ethics was taught to them. Almost invariably the reply is that there was little or no formal teaching of ethics. But then a curious anecdote will emerge, which will suggest something about the kind of standards to which physicians somehow learn to conform. In Belgium, for example, physicians are expected not to get drunk in public; even in nonmedical situations, physicians are expected to maintain different standards of conduct. In Ghana, a physician was censored by the medical society for getting into an altercation with a taxi driver about the fee, suggesting that physicians should be so dedicated to service of others that any attempt to stand up for their own interests reflects badly on the profession. In Sweden, physicians understand that they should not accept presents from a patient, unless it is a small token like a potholder, but not something as valuable as a lobster. In the United States, the owner of a riding stable complained that a physician was "unethical" (that is, "unprofessional") because of rudeness in a dispute about riding time. The physician was reprimanded by the professional society, not for standing up for his rights, but for identifying himself as a physician in the dispute.

These examples may sound quixotic, but they serve to illustrate the range of issues that may be considered under the heading of "medical ethics." It may be useful therefore to keep in mind the differing tasks of ethics, which may lead to different methods of ethical reflection depending on one's purposes. The maintaining of clear distinctions about the tasks of ethics may help to eliminate some of the confusion that arises when the various approaches to

47

ethics seem to be at cross-purposes. In the interest of maintaining that clarity, I offer the comparisons sketched in Figure 1.

The upward perspective is that *of* the individual agent in relation to the larger culture. The downward perspective is the view *on* the individual from the perspective of the norms of the culture or group. In what I call the "upward perspective," we are talking about the very highest standards of ethical conduct to which anyone might aspire—ethical ideals, not moral imperatives. The task of ethics in the downward perspective is regulation of abuse. In terms of a profession, this would be the profession "policing itself," if viewed from within the profession, or subjecting the profession to scrutiny, if viewed from without. The upward perspective is that of the individual (practitioner) seeking to insure that his or her own conduct is the highest possible. The upward perspective presupposes the mutual trust of the physician and patient in their collaboration. There is no maximal limit on mutual responsibility of the patient and physician in their partnership. But there are minimal limits. The downward perspective is that of the regulatory agency or professional society seeking to insure that the behavior of a particular individual does not fall below certain minimal standards. No trust is assumed, and in the downward perspective ambiguity is reduced through an adversarial procedure such as peer review, Institutional Review Board (IRB), or actual judicial process.

These two approaches to ethics are not mutually exclusive, nor do they demand that one choose between them. Rather they serve very different purposes, operating at times simultaneously in the minds of a given person or group as a way of getting beyond the habits of modern thought that would have us choose *either* one *or* the other when both are needed.

❦ *Figure 1. The Tasks of Ethics*

Upward Perspective	**Downward Perspective**
Moral Inspiration	Regulation of abuse
Affective	Cognitive
Self-reflective	Critical
Post-critical	Analytical
Teleological (end-based, goal-based)	Deontological (rule-based)
Fiduciary relationship (based on trust)	Adversary relationship (based on control)
Tacit	Explicit

The recognition of multiple tasks of ethics, as disclosed by considering the operative norms of special groups such as the medical profession, raises questions not only about how one chooses among conflicting allegiances, but also about how to understand what one is about when "doing" ethics. When is a question or issue to be understood as an ethical question or issue? Does it depend on one's perspective? If so, does this suggest that different conclusions could be reached in different situations? If not, could one hope for an absolute guideline as a point of reference in making decisions? Our task will be to look at what we can learn about our culture from the ways in which we apply moral principles to particular situations.

William Frankena, in his practical and popular text, *Ethics,* distinguishes two philosophical theories of moral obligation, *teleological* and *deontological* ethical theories.[8]

Teleological ethical theories

Teleogical ethical theories (from the Greek *telos,* meaning end or goal) hold that the ultimate standard by which an act is judged morally right, wrong, obligatory, or correct is the general happiness of all people concerned, or the greatest net balance of good over evil. This is often identified as the principle of utility or beneficence, which implies that good and bad are capable of being measured and balanced against each other in some quantitative or mathematical way. ("The greatest good for the greatest number.") Thus teleological theories often go by the name of *utilitarianism*. They are represented by such philosophers as Jeremy Bentham, John Stuart Mill, G. E. Moore, and more recently by Joseph Fletcher, whose situation ethics employs as its central principle "agape," the love for humanity, or general goodwill. . . . It should be noted, of course, that not all teleologists are utilitarians. Plato, Augustine, and even Aristotle all strove to articulate principles of conduct, but would be horrified by the mathematical connotations of "utilitarianism."

Act-utilitarians judge each action individually according to whether it will promote the general happiness, whereas *rule-utilitarians* select rules of conduct that are judged to promote the general happiness and then act in accordance with those rules. Figure 2 illustrates in a schematic algorithm (decision tree) the steps involved in the act-utilitarian form of the teleological ethical method.[10] This visual schema depicts the variable dimension of time as well as the necessity for mathematical quantification. The decision-making process starts with a perception of a problem and proceeds to a listing of all the conceivable alternatives, for which consequences are predicted and values of happiness assigned. The limitations of this method are that the method fails if one is unable to predict the consequences accurately or if one is unable to estimate accurate happiness values. In medical ethical dilemmas, it is often difficult to predict consequences accurately. For example, it was generally assumed Karen Quinlan would die if her respirator were turned off; she did not. Furthermore, there is often such a disparity between the individual happiness or suffering and the general social welfare that it makes it very difficult to calculate happiness values in individual situations. What and whose happiness is being considered when a respirator is turned off? Our awesome ambivalence in the face of death makes it difficult even to acknowledge consciously the full range of alternatives and their possible consequences. What might be the real impact of such things as elective death, suicide, and euthanasia, both active and passive, and how close are they psychologically to murder?

Figure 2.   Act-Utilitarian Ethical Method

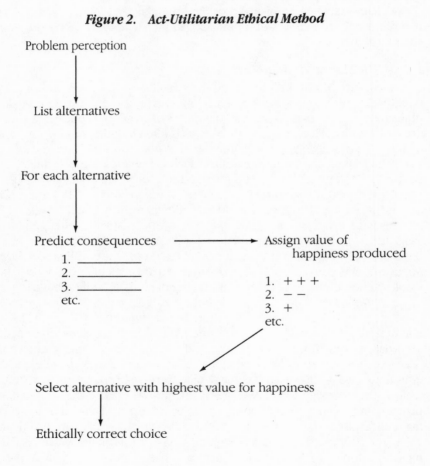

Problem perception

List alternatives

For each alternative

Predict consequences   ⟶   Assign value of
   1. _____   happiness produced
   2. _____
   3. _____   1. + + +
   etc.   2. − −
                     3. +
                     etc.

Select alternative with highest value for happiness

Ethically correct choice

Method fails if:
   1. Unable to predict consequences accurately
   2. Unable to estimate happiness values

Deontological ethical theories

Deontological ethical theories maintain that there are rules or principles of action that have moral validity independent of the consequences and that one must act in accordance with these rules or principles. Deontological theories assert that there are considerations other than goodness or badness on which decisions are to be based, things such as keeping a promise, maintaining justice, or adhering to a commandment of God or the state, which are important regardless of the consequences of the action. One finds deontological theories in well-defined communities, such as religious communities, where one of the ethical considerations is preservation of the social order. Professional standards of ethics have such deontological features, where the rule or principle may be applied to exclude or coerce the deviant member to maintain the reputation of the group. Duty, obligation, obedience, and loyalty are the values that define deontological functioning. Because of the specificity of the application of ethical principles and the possibility of conflict among principles, principles or laws tend to be elaborated to apply to various situations. Thus one sees the development of a complex corpus of law and devoted study as in Talmudic scholarship or in American constitutional law. This problem can be avoided in ethical theory if one can claim that only one basic principle exists. The best example of this kind of pure rule deontology is Immanuel Kant's categorical imperative, which in its first form states, "Act only on that maxim which you can at the same time will to be a universal law,"[11] or alternatively stated, "Act always so as to treat people as ends and not merely as means only."[12]

Figure 3 delineates the steps in decision making by the deontological ethical method. The alternative actions arising from a perceived problem are compared with a list of rules or principles. If there is no consistency, one may appeal to a higher authority in search of a right action. However, one is left unguided if the rule or principle (or authority) does not specify action in a particular situation or if the application or rules or principles results in conflict.

An example of a case in which Kant's principle might be illuminating is the question of removing an organ from a "brain-dead" person on a respirator for transplantation. By the notion that brain function is necessary for "personhood," the body is not a person, and we are free to use it as a means toward some other valued end: saving someone else's life. But we are similarly not free to save another's life by removing an organ from a living person without his consent; that would be using the person as a means and not as an end in himself. Under strict utilitarian guidelines, we could do so if the general happiness would be increased—for example, if the person needing the organ was a great scientist and the involuntary donor was a depraved criminal. Here the Kantian deontologist could claim his method to be superior to utilitarianism, because it attributes to the individual not just value, which is relative, but the dignity of being regarded as an end in himself.

Figure 3. Deontological Ethical Method

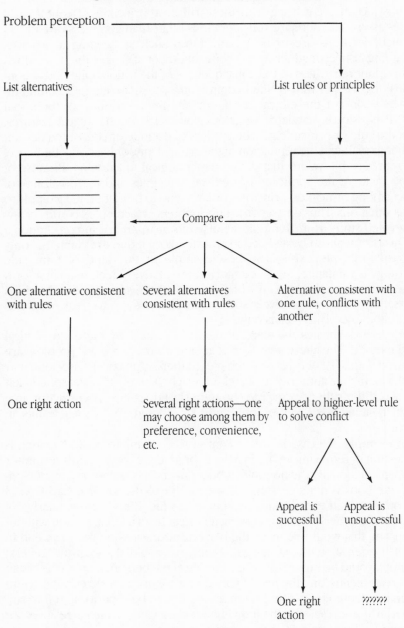

The teleological and deontological ethical methods share as liabilities the abstractness of their application. By attempting to dissect for analysis the ingredients involved in decision making, many considerations that cannot be easily articulated or brought to consciousness fail to receive sufficient attention. Cognitive elements are stressed while affective elements may be suppressed.

The consequentialist approach

Another method of ethical reasoning is the *consequentialist* approach, a method by which an action is judged to be morally right or wrong by assessing the consequences of the action. Utilitarianism is in fact a form of consequentialist ethics inasmuch as it specifies criteria, such as general happiness, by which moral actions are to be judged.

The consequentialist ethical method is diagrammed in Figure 4. Several features immediately distinguished this method from the teleological and deontological methods . For example, one of the first steps is to make a choice among the alternatives—before reflection and analysis. This accounts for the human tendency to favor a particular course of action at a "gut level," which is not necessarily wrong so long as those inclinations are carefully scrutinized. The feedback loops in Figure 4 account for that process of consideration and reconsideration. The consequentialist method accounts for cognitive factors in its demand for consistency as a test of the validity of a given ethical statement. What is striking is that the method also recognizes the affective components and insists that they too be considered. The short test might be paraphrased as "Is this an action I could be comfortable with?" It properly gives attention to affective as well as cognitive considerations.

The striking contrast between the consequentialist and the absolutist methods is the consequentialist focus on personal considerations as the deciding factors and the absolutist focus on the issues, independent of personal considerations. One might immediately say "Of course, these are not mutually exclusive alternatives; one need consider *both* the deciding agent *and* the issue." The matter would be simple were it not for the altogether too familiar experience we have all had in ethical arguments, bull sessions, or political debate of seeing relevant personal issues discounted as meaninglessly subjective and therefore unworthy of consideration in an argument tacitly governed by a demand for total explicitness and impersonality. This experience of impotent frustration suggests some of the sources of social discontent of the poor, the weak, and the powerless in calling moral attention to their situation. What kinds of arguments can be advanced that have suasion over the social order? Though such dynamics are complex, we must at least consider their implications for ethical theory.

Recently theologians such as Stanley Hauerwas and philosophers such as Edmund Pincoffs have attacked the absolutist view of ethics, which holds that ethics should deduce by reason a truth that could be applied in a particular

Figure 4.   *Consequentialist Ethical Method*

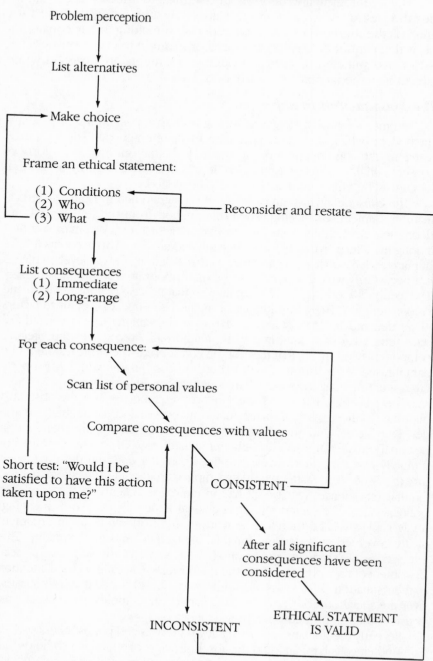

dilemma. This view, Hauerwas points out, holds that ethics should be universal, impersonal, atemporal, and acultural. Hauerwas contrasts this standard account with an approach based on "story" or narrative to reemphasize the centrality of the moral agent in moral action. His critique hinges on a view of "objectivity" at work in modern culture that contaminates thinking about ethics by requireing a dissociation between the issue and the agent, the truth and the knower of the truth, the decision and the decider. About this notion of objectivity and its deleterious consequences for our moral life, I have more to say in the following chapters, but Hauerwas very deftly sets the tone in the context of our consideration of ethical theory.

> I am not trying to supplement the Kantian paradigm that appears to many today to be the only intelligible form of moral objectivity; rather I am trying to provide a new way to conceive of moral rationality and objectivity. It is not the demand for "objective moral judgements" that has misled us, but rather the theories of "objectivity" that have dominated the modern period.[13]

Hauerwas specifically takes exception to Frankena's approach to ethics, which attempts to explain ethical behavior in terms of a theory of obligation, rather than adequately accounting for the notion of "virtue" in explaining why people are moral. The critique is an important one because among the moral philosophers, Frankena does recognize the importance of the concept of virtue for moral life, but he seems unable to divorce himself sufficiently from the standard objectivist account to give an adequately developed moral psychology. For example, he notes that when one turns from the "vivid accounts of human life and action" found in Shakespeare to moral philosophy, the latter seems remote and abstract from the facts of life.[14] This confession may reveal the predicament of the moral philosopher, who in his account of moral theory in a rigorously objective fashion is reluctant to mess with the uncertainties and ambiguities that accompany subjectivity. This realization is not to devalue the importance of a well-grounded theory of moral obligation, but rather to open up for consideration the more personal, but less precisely specifiable, elements of moral life. Put starkly in Hauerwas's words, "Integrity, not obligation, is the hallmark of the moral life."[15] Integrity is literally an integration of our beliefs about the world in which we live and our beliefs about the values and purposes by which we should conduct our lives. Integrity includes (but is not limited to) obligation to externally conceived imperatives. More fundamentally it issues from internal commitments, which we honor to maintain our sense of who we are. It is a psychosomatic integrity of mind (thoughts) and bodily feelings (affects).

This approach to ethics may seem so obvious as to be trivial and at the same time so threatening as to require strenuous denunciation. To consider an approach to ethics that is not universal—but rather personal, temporal, and cultural—raises the spectre of ethical relativism. To admit psychological consideration into ethical reflection raises the possibility of pluralism and individualism, which might threaten the social stability. To consider personal motives, intentions, and emotions may seem tantamount to opening Pandora's Box. Nietzsche's observation that "If God is dead, anything is permitted," may be paraphrased, "If science is not heeded in ethics, anything may be permitted." Abraham Edel, in considering the uses of science in ethics, notes that "traditionally morality rested on supernaturalist or non-naturalist bases," meaning "an absolute moral order founded on a religious framework." However, "the growth of science and technology in modern times, with their vast accompanying changes in mode of life, ushered in a secular atmosphere."[16] Recognizing the possibility of relative values (that is, recognizing the possibility that someone might counter an absolutist approach with "It all depends . . ."), Edel turns to the "human sciences"—biology, psychology, anthropology, sociology, and history—in search of a "common ethic." Science then is asked to provide what religion no longer can; that is, a compelling basis for ethics. Michael Scriven also appeals for a scientific approach to ethics and is equally distraught at the possibility of irrationality in ethics: "It is stupefying to realize that a generation of philosophers was content to accept the idea that there could not be good reasons for morality."[17]

Scriven's outburst has an intimidating quality to it. For anyone schooled in the dominant modes of Western philosophy and modern thought who cannot immediately articulate these "good reasons for morality," Scriven's remark evokes almost shameful defensiveness. Even though careful reflection does not in fact yield good prescriptive norms or suggest their application in practice, one gets the feeling that one should seek this sort of articulation. Indeed it would seem almost heretical—should one say unscientific?—to suggest that moral actions do not in fact issue from reflected, abstracted, conscious, philosophical positions, but rather issue from the considered judgment of moral agents and reflect values formed over a lifetime of commitments.

Thus in questioning the methods of ethics, no less a question than the methods of science and their relationship to ethics must be considered. Furthermore, the relationship of religion and science must be considered, for it is an oversimplification to say scientific thinking has supplanted religious thinking in the modern age. Modern scientific thought had its origins in religious philosophy, and it is the way in which these two modes of thought came to be separated that characterizes the modern age. The crisis for ethics—and more particularly the crisis of confidence faced by modern medicine—must be understood by appreciating the outlook that requires us to choose between either matters of fact or matters of value.

It is precisely the question "What is ethics all about?" that characterizes the modern age. In some fields, but not ethics, it is fashionable to speak of one period or another as an age, characterized by certain values, a certain style, and a certain worldview. In ethics, one searches for timeless values, which should transcend the whims of a particular generation. Our time is often considered unique because of the special problems it presents for ethics by virtue of its manifold technological innovations. The modern age does pose some special challenges, not just in locating the eternal verities in a maze of technological innovations, but in the very process of examining ethics. Ours is a time when moral argument is not only unfashionable but also almost alien to the characteristic modes of intellectual thought and social discourse—yet paradoxically a time that, though we may be reluctant to admit it, is intensely and perfectionistically moral, as we shall have an opportunity to consider in later chapters.

CHAPTER 4

CONFIDENTIALITY, TRUST, AND THE THERAPEUTIC ALLIANCE

T HE PRINCIPLE OF CONFIDENTIALITY is one of the central features of all professions. It is a requirement of anyone working intimately with others seeking help. It is the cornerstone of any group that considers itself professional. Doctors, lawyers, and clergy—the paradigm professions—all take confidentiality with utmost seriousness, as do psychotherapists and counselors, bankers, and accountants. The work of the professional requires the guarantee of secrecy. Without it, professional work could not take place. Without it, we could not turn to another and disclose our needs for help.

Yet the ability to guarantee secrecy in a professional relationship is not easily achieved or maintained. There are always pressures on the professional to divulge what is disclosed in confidence. There are always others who claim an interest in what people share in professional relationships. Sometimes the interests are legitimate "for the societal good," and the professional may experience an ethical tension between his promise to maintain secrecy and some competing claim for attention. Physicians have readily come to accept the legitimacy of insurance companies wanting to know something about the treatments they are paying for. Lawyers are placed in conflict between their clients and society when criminal activities are disclosed. Psychiatrists and other psychotherapists may experience a similar conflict when they suspect a patient may intend to harm another.

For the medical profession, the idea of protecting confidences goes back to the Hippocratic Oath, which states,

> And whatsoever I shall see or hear in the course of my profession, as well as outside my profession in my intercourse with men, if it be what should not be published abroad, I will never divulge, holding such things to be holy secrets.

It is worth noting that the Hippocratic Oath leaves much to the discretion of the physician. The physician must judge what should not be published abroad.

The notion of confidentiality recurs in almost all codes of professional ethics. It is part of the Declaration of Geneva. It was a central part of Percival's *Medical Ethics* (1803), which formed the basis of both the AMA's first code of medical ethics in 1847 and subsequent revisions as well as the British Medical Association's codes of medical ethics.

The legal protection of confidentiality comes much later but also has a venerable standing. It has been part of English common law since the seventeenth century. In 1606 Guy Fawkes planned to assassinate the capricious King James I by blowing up Parliament, the famous "gunpowder plot." He confessed his plans to his priest, who was later hanged for treason when the plot was uncovered. Later priests and then lawyers were given the protection of confidentiality under law. British physicians still do not enjoy the legal protection of confidentiality, but physicians in most countries do. Some places, like California, also extend that protection to nonmedical psychotherapists.

THE NEED FOR CONFIDENTIALITY

For psychotherapists especially, but no less so for all physicians, trust is essential for the healing process. The patient must trust the physician in order to disclose intimate concerns. This we appreciate. But even more important, trust is essential for healing to take place in ways we do not fully understand. We have long spoken of the importance of trust in the doctor-patient relationship. We can imagine in Hippocratic times the physician might have little more to offer than hope, inspiration, and a healthful spa-like environment. We might seriously ask if these less-tangible ingredients still have a legitimate place in medicine when so much can be accomplished by physiological intervention.

Nowadays when one speaks of the medical model, it is usually understood that the medical model implies a biological reductionistic model, the doctor's role being to correct some abnormality of physiological functioning through pharmacological or surgical intervention. History taking may not seem particularly important beyond a declaration of symptoms because diagnosis may be made by biochemical test or radiological imaging.

This is obviously a deviation from the Hippocratic tradition in medicine with its ethical emphasis on the centrality of confidentiality in the doctor-patient relationship. Although there are many who would say that the Hippocratic Oath is obsolete because it provides little guidance in dealing with modern technology, I would suggest just the opposite. It is the ethical traditions that define medicine and provide a human context for the application of technology.

THREATS TO CONFIDENTIALITY

A physician schooled in the traditions of professional ethics takes the issue of the patient's confidence with utmost seriousness. But there are also competing demands made by society upon the professional's allegiance. The professional is often asked to serve not only the patient or client but society as well. There are numerous situations that threaten not only the privilege of the doctor-patient (or professional-client) relationship, but the very existence of the professions as professions.

I will now suggest a number of areas of conflict between the professional's interest in maintaining the secrecy of privileged communications and the demands placed upon the professional by society imposing or attempting to impose interests of its own. In each of the cases it is possible to see the immediate need of society in the claims made upon the professional to override confidentiality. The issue of trust lurking behind the principle is sometimes less obvious and may therefore require some reconsideration in light of the larger question of professional definition and the importance to society of protecting the relationship implied in a professional covenant.

The Tarasoff case: protecting public safety

The *Tarasoff* decision is widely discussed as a threat to confidentiality. An alarming decision by the California Supreme Court, *Tarasoff* involves the state's willingness to use the therapist as its own agent when the patient/client appears likely to harm an identifiable third party. It is argued that protecting public safety is the rationale for overriding confidentiality.

The facts of the case are as follows: Prosenjit Poddar, a student at the University of California at Berkeley, fell in love and became obsessed with a young woman named Tatiana Tarasoff. His love was unrequited; he became depressed and underwent counseling at the Student Health Services. His therapist became alarmed and reported him to the University police, who questioned Poddar and warned him to stay away from Tatiana, but they did not apply for emergency evaluation and treatment applicable under California's involuntary hospitalization laws. Poddar broke off treatment—the confidentiality already violated—and several months later murdered Tatiana. Her parents sued the therapist, the police, and the regents of the university, on the grounds that they had a duty to protect Tatiana from Poddar.

The California Supreme Court concluded that therapists, but not the police, have a duty to warn a potential victim since they have a special relationship with the potentially dangerous person. The court noted that "the protective privilege ends where the public peril begins."[1]

The *Tarasoff* decision is particularly bad because it weakens the legal protection of confidentiality for reasons that will probably accomplish very little. The real issue in the *Tarasoff* case is not confidentiality or even the prediction of violence, but the extreme emphasis on individual liberties and the difficulty in utilizing civil commitment procedures. Although most therapists would probably compromise confidentiality in the likely event of imminent physical danger—as did Poddar's therapist—the disclosure of the threat in itself does little to protect the would-be victim. The real issue is the taking away of one person's civil liberties through involuntary hospitalization when those liberties threaten the existence of someone else. The *Tarasoff* decision does not address these crucial issues. Warning potential victims then gives them the responsibility for protecting themselves, a responsibility that the state had abdicated. Indeed the *Tarasoff* decision is really a testimony to social indifference and anonymity in an urban community. Tatiana Tarasoff's murder was tragic; the *Tarasoff* decision reduces the situation to melodrama.

Preventing fraud: review of MEDICARE records

Prevention of fraud is the rationale for requiring review of Medicare and other health care records. This practice is so extensive and so many people have access to health records that very little true privacy is left in health care.

While patients usually give a blanket consent for these reviews, such consent cannot be truly considered an informed consent in the sense of a free, uncoerced choice, for the patient has little choice if faced with loss of coverage. It is true that many people choose not to use insurance coverage for psychotherapy and other services, but this is a luxury not everyone can afford.

Furthermore, the patient may make disclosures to the physician, trusting his or her confidences to someone trained to elicit them and ethically bound to protect them. There is of course no such ethical standard governing the multitude of clerks and reviewers who may then gain access to some or all of the information so disclosed.

Aware of this feature of the contemporary medical record, most physicians of necessity limit what is included in the written reports. The patient may report any number of intimacies that are then either not included in the record or merely alluded to, thereby diminishing the value of the record for those directly involved in patient care or for those who might subsequently attempt to do retrospective research from the medical record.

Even more serious is the possibility that the patient, aware of the widespread circulation of records, will choose not to confide details that might be relevant and therefore limit the quality of care that might otherwise be available.

Here we witness the kind of erosion of trust that undermines not only the quality of health care, but also the human quality of our social institutions as well. What starts out as an apparently legitimate interest in protecting against fraud ultimately brings about an increasingly suspicious and self-protective society.

Redisclosure in information banks

Information disclosed to physicians and duly recorded in the medical record can be reviewed by insurance companies under the ostensible reason of protecting against fraud and then redisclosed for other purposes through massive computer information banks. Neither the patient who consented to disclosure nor the physician need be aware of the uses to which this information might be put. So widespread is the practice and so far is it from the privacy of the doctor's office that legislative vigilance is really in order. Perhaps some sort of specific consent for each redisclosure of information should be required.

Cost containment and using the physician as an agent of rationing health care

If there is any feature of health economics that has been widely recognized it is the high cost of medical care and the need to limit health costs. For more than a decade now, "cost consciousness" has been a byword of medical education and public debate. The physician, as the most immediate spender of the health care dollar, has been expected to lower this burden on the national economy. To the extent that economies could be achieved by increased efficiency—that is, eliminating waste and redundancy by such things as foregoing unnecessary testing—this movement poses no conflict with professional ethics. But when the physician is asked to be the agent of rationing at the bedside by limiting potentially beneficial care given to a particular patient, he or she is placed in a conflict of interest situation *vis à vis* that particular patient. Ethically that physician might be required to issue a Miranda-like warning: "Trust me, but be aware that I will do as little for you as economically possible."

Prearraignment examinations

In several cities it is common practice to employ psychiatrists to interview criminal suspects in the jails before they are arraigned. Information so obtained may later be used as evidence at trial. The APA Ethics Committee has raised serious questions about this practice as a violation of the confidentiality requirement of the code of ethics all members agree to follow. Psychiatrists are so employed because they are good at eliciting information. Techniques used to promote trust and elicit disclosure for the purpose of helping the person can also be used in the interests of society against that person. The message, "Trust me—I would like to be of help to you" can be abridged simply to "Trust me," but such activity is clearly beyond the ethical scope of the professional's obligation to the patient. If professionals agree to participate in such activities, they must make very clear to those they are interviewing/interrogating what the purpose of the investigation really is.

Advancing scientific knowledge: case reports

Advancing scientific knowledge through case reports is one of the reasons that is sometimes suggested for compromising confidentiality and disclosing information gained in the course of treatment, particularly in psychotherapy or psychoanalysis. It is never ethical to disclose information about a patient in such a way that the identity of the person might be recognized by others. But how much disguise is adequate? And is it necessary to obtain explicit consent from the patient to publish or present case material?

These are issues of interest both for the establishment of professional standards and for the courts. Because of a number of judgments against psychiatrists or psychologists for inadequate disguise, we have witnessed a marked reduction in the number of case reports in the literature. Indeed we are increasingly likely to see statistical studies of populations, rather than in-depth studies of individuals. Consequently, focus on the individual person may receive less attention in treatment as well as in research.

This would suggest that there is indeed a legitimate place for the case report as a way of preserving the human focus on the individual patient. So how can the educational and scientific need for awareness of what goes on in the office of the experienced psychotherapist be balanced against the need to protect confidentiality?

Certainly historical and biographical details can be sufficiently altered or disguised to protect the patient's identity, focusing in the presentation on dynamic details, course of treatment, resistances, transference, and such matters. Explicit consent is desirable from an ethical point of view if it could be obtained without distorting the course of the therapy. But if disguise is adequate, explicit consent should not be necessary unless the presentation involved videotaped materials that would make disguise impossible. In such cases consent should be obtained not only for the taping of sessions or interviews, but with specific permission for each showing and audience.

Professional gossip

Professional gossip falls in a category by itself. It is perhaps one of the most serious threats to confidentiality for which one cannot suggest that there is any competing societal interest that would legitimately justify the disclosure. Instead the compromise of confidentiality is motivated by psychological needs of the therapist to disclose for personal reasons. If one has a celebrity patient, there may be a strong urge to let others know to enhance one's own self-esteem and perhaps to enhance referrals. This is the sort of situation that professional review should monitor most seriously, for such capricious disclosure compromises not only the care that individual receives, but diminishes the reputation of the professional group as well.

Similarly psychiatrists may be asked to comment on public figures. Presidents and presidential candidates are often sources of much curiosity about whom a psychiatrist could say a great deal, but must not. When Barry Goldwater was running for president, over one thousand psychiatrists responded to a magazine questionnaire offering "professional opinions" about his mental health, much to the embarrassment of their profession and ultimately themselves. It is unethical to offer a professional opinion if one has not examined the patient, and if one has examined the patient, it is unethical to publicly disclose that opinion without proper authorization.

Psychohistory is another example in which the research psychiatrist might be tempted to publicly comment upon the details of a famous figure's personal life. Such disclosures are subject to judgment of two kinds of professional standards, the confidentiality requirements of the professional group and also the scholarly standards for research of this sort in terms of the genuine contribution to knowledge.

At a personal level, one should always scrutinize one's motives for disclosure: Is it for genuine enhancement of knowledge or for personal aggrandizement? But one also needs to recognize that such disclosures are also regulated by codes of professional standards as well as legal standards, the distinction made in Chapter 2 between the upward and downward perspectives of ethical functioning.

Access to records by patients

The question often arises, "Who owns the medical record?" Should the physician disclose to the patient the contents of the medical record? This might seem a curious question in an analysis of confidentiality since it is a question of the physician keeping the patient's secret a secret from the patient. However, the question of promoting trust puts the issue in perspective. The physician should be guided by the principle of promoting the patient's confidence. Practically this means disclosing to the patient not only what the patient has revealed, but also the physician's judgments. Legally the patient has the right to make that claim, though it may require time-consuming court action. The disclosure may not be an instantaneous and impersonal release of the records but rather an ongoing dialogue about what one knows and is finding. The question usually would not arise unless there was some cause for suspicion or conflict between the doctor and patient. That could mean "retentiveness" or unnecessary withholding on the part of the physician or undue suspicion or paranoia on the part of the patient.

Treating the same person in both individual and group therapy

If a particular therapist is treating the same individual in both individual and group therapy, can that therapist ethically disclose to the group information that is disclosed in the individual sessions? Such a disclosure would obviously be a violation of confidentiality in the private relationship and as such highlights the tension between the commitment to the individual and the group or "larger society." A similar issue involves the treatment of an individual and a couple by the same therapist. The fact that the question arises so often suggests the dynamic difficulties of trying to balance such conflicting allegiances, the interests of the individual and those of the group. Secrets in such a context can be used as a tool for manipulation or as a weapon to covertly express hostility. The motives need to be clarified and interpreted. It would obviously be an oversimplification to suggest that one therapist should not have the same patient in both individual or group therapy, but it should be appreciated that discharging one's professional responsibilities under such circumstances may be difficult. Confidences can be violated only at peril.

Psychiatric testimony in custody cases

The psychiatrist treating one or another parties in a divorce may be called into court to testify about custody matters. Should he or she disclose what is learned in therapy sessions? Must such information be disclosed to the court? The ethical questions and the legal question cut in slightly different ways. Ethically the psychiatrist is bound to secrecy and should refuse to disclose what is learned, but the court may require a disclosure in its interest in making a suitable determination. There are many famous cases of psychiatrists cited for contempt of court in such situations for refusing to testify.[2] Should the psychiatrist find himself in such a conflict, he should be very hesitant to take the interest of the state against the interest of his patient without making it very clear that testimony is given only at the requirement of the court. In such situations review and consent of the patient should also be obtained.

Nonprofessionals on health care teams

In a psychiatric hospital or ward or even working in a family situation, the treating psychiatrist may work with nonprofessionals or family helpers who do not share the same professional respect for confidentiality. In such situations the psychiatrist should not assume others working with the patient will respect the same standards of confidentiality. Rather the psychiatrist must make a judgment about what, if anything, needs to be disclosed and make sure to review with other caregivers what standards of confidentiality are expected.

Similarly in working with family members, it cannot be assumed that relatives of a patient will bear that patient's interest ahead of their own. They may make claims upon the physician's allegiance that might run counter to the best interests of the patient. In such situations where cooperation of family is essential, it is part of the physician's Hippocratic commitment to the patient to attempt to involve families members in the therapeutic alliance.

Mandatory reporting of suspected child abuse

Even more distressing than the *Tarasoff* decision from the standpoint of confidentiality are the new laws requiring mandatory reporting of suspected child abuse. While the *Tarasoff* decision sacrifices the protection of confidentiality for a compelling interest of the state, the unusual and extreme circumstances are ones that might well force one to compromise confidentiality anyway. The mandatory reporting statutes, however worthy the intent of protecting children, require reporting in circumstances that may make ongoing therapy impossible. Furthermore, the mandatory reporting statutes may adversely alter the lives of the people involved since the only tool available to the state is to separate the members of a family, which may be an even more damaging trauma.

Today all 50 states as well as the District of Columbia and the territories have laws requiring clinicians of various professional disciplines to report any instance of known or "reasonably suspected" child abuse to a "child protective agency." Child abuse includes any "unjustifiable mental suffering," a variety of specific and general sexual behaviors, and the usual acts of physical injury, cruelty, and neglect. These laws require an immediate report (usually the requirement is of an immediate telephone report followed within 36 hours by a written report) without the opportunity to exercise professional judgment regarding either the appropriateness or the implications of doing so. The government agencies are given the function of deciding how to investigate and intervene. Failure to report leaves the clinician vulnerable to criminal as well as civil prosecution. Only two states, Maryland and Maine, allow the professional the discretion *not* to report.[3]

The effects of these overreaching laws are increasingly familiar to psychiatrists as well as to other physicians and mental health workers. Many have experienced professional dilemmas such as whether to report a parent who comes to therapy concerned about how to discipline an unruly child or concerned about sexual fantasies or impulses he is not always able to control.

A Chapel Hill psychologist was convicted on criminal charges of failing to report suspected child abuse, fined $200, and given a suspended sentence. Parents of two adopted children, a boy 13 and a girl 10, came to the psychologist for help in disciplining the children. When spankings failed, they had resorted to "timing the children out" in their basement, sometimes for several days at a time. The children were fed and allowed to go the bathroom. Prior to a determination of whether these actions actually constituted abuse, the children were removed from the home by the police, thus adding to their traumatic cycle of separation and loss.[4]

Another example of this sort of nightmare is a much-reported San Francisco case:

Twelve-year old "Amy" reported to her mother that her stepfather (a physician) was fondling her. When her mother became convinced of the truth of the matter, she required that her husband move out of the house for the time being and that both parents and Amy seek professional help for their problems. The counselor, in compliance with the California law, duly informed the local child protective agency. The parents were stripped of custody, and the district attorney filed charges against the stepfather.

Amy repeatedly refused to testify against her stepfather, whereupon the judge found her guilty of contempt and ordered her held in a four-by-eight windowless, solitary confinement cell. When Amy again declined to testify after five days of punitive confinement, the judge ordered her held over the weekend and barred further visits from her mother. Only after eight days was Amy's attorney able to obtain a release from a superior court judge, and she was transferred to a foster home. Finally Amy was made a ward of the court, and returned to her mother. The stepfather was ordered not to see Amy, and the family was ordered to undergo treatment. The mother and stepfather continued to live in separation, reportedly trying to work out a reconciliation.[5]

The horrors of child abuse inspire people to action and there can be little question that the mandatory reporting laws are well intended. But they are ill conceived. The venerable and somewhat creaky principle of confidentiality does not inspire the same kind of fervent action, but it must be carefully protected so that the kind of trusting, intimate relationships and self-disclosure that might effect changes can take place. Clearly legislative reform is in order, and one need only cite the Maryland and Maine statutes with their provisions *not* to report as examples of the kind of reform necessary. It might be too much to expect that courts will conduct themselves in a more "professional" manner. Given the tension between the emotionally charged confrontations of the courtroom and the more personal attention of the professional relationship, it does not seem unreasonable to expect some professional stewardship allowing for a more individualized approach.

THE DOUBLE AGENT PROBLEM

In all of these examples we see a conflict between the commitment of the professional to the person served and some other claim on the professional's allegiance. This conflict is sometimes called the "double agent problem." The classic example of the double agent problem is the psychiatrist working for the military, treating patients also working for his employer. In time of war, the psychiatrist's job may be to get his patients psychologically fit to go back to battle and risk their lives, hopefully for the good of their country (that is, the common good). However, the conflict of interest may not always involve such noble considerations.

At a lecture I gave on confidentiality, a physician in the audience related the following story from his experience as a medical officer during the Korean War: A soldier reported to the infirmary with feelings of depression and an inability to sleep, eat, or concentrate on his work. He said he was upset because his homosexual lover had rejected him. He expressed thoughts of suicide. The physician referred the soldier to a nearby psychiatric unit. There the admitting officer met the soldier, not with the usual offer to help, but with the announcement that this would mean an end to the soldier's military career. Shortly after that the soldier shot and killed himself.

While the military offers dramatic examples of double agentry, the problem is increasingly widespread. Any physician working for a corporation, a health maintenance organization, or another prepayment plan intended to reduce care given to an individual patient, or any physician working for a government under a socialized payment system (in short, anyone not working directly for the patient), must wrestle with the double agent problem. The only way it can be successfully addressed is by being constantly mindful of it. It is one of the functions of professional ethics to keep those reminders alive through education, codes, and professional discipline.

LEGAL PERSPECTIVES ON THE ETHICAL PRINCIPLE

Several distinctions need to be made. First of all is the distinction between privacy and confidentiality. Privacy applies to individuals. It is the patient/client who controls access and disclosure of information in the first instance. Once that information is disclosed to the professional, confidentiality applies. Confidentiality is a concept that applies only to relationships.

We also need to distinguish between legal standards and ethical standards. They are different and their goals are different. Legal decisions are frozen in time; they are static. They isolate the moment of choice apart from history. Ethical decisions are dynamic and fraught with ongoing tension. They involve relationships in families and communities that endure in time. They involve not just isolated instances, but also the development of character, the kind of people we choose to be or strive to become and the kind of society we wish to be.

Confidentiality is the domain of ethics; it involves relationships. If we see the professional's job as trying to balance the interests of the state with those of the patient/client, it is clear that the state can bring a lot of weight to bear on its side. But this is where the professional culture can also bring some weight to bear.

The concept of confidentiality is so essential to professional life that we cannot exist *as professionals* without it. Therefore, when asked or pressured to divulge confidences, we do not do so easily because it is not just a particular relationship that is threatened, but our professional selves.

If we look at the tension between society and our patients or clients, I think the concept of the therapeutic alliance might be helpful in mediating the tension. The alliance is the partnership that makes disclosure and working together possible. It requires confidentiality, which promotes trust.

Trust is important not just to gain information, but as a healing element in itself. Therefore, if we look for an overriding principle by which a particular conflict might be resolved, we could say that promoting and protecting trust is the goal at both an individual level and at the level of social policy.

Let me use one case to illustrate, the case of Dr. R. J. D. Browne:

> *Dr. Browne was charged with improperly disclosing to the father of a girl then aged 16 that she had been prescribed an oral contraceptive by the Birmingham Brook Advisory Center. In a* British Medical Journal *editorial the dismissal of the charges against Dr. Browne by the General Medical Council Disciplinary Committee was hailed as a triumphant reaffirmation of "the principles of medical*

practice that the doctor has an obligation to act in the way he judges to be in the best interests of his patient."[6]

But what about the fiduciary principle of a trusting partnership? If this 16-year-old girl got pregnant, could she then turn to Dr. Browne with the expectation of help? The principle of independence of the doctor's clinical judgment only makes sense if the doctor is prepared to weigh the tradeoffs when principles conflict with the trust-promoting considerations of an ongoing relationship. What did this girl need? How might her doctor have helped her?

Clearly Dr. Browne needed some sense of a cooperative partnership with his patient, a working alliance. Eventually he might even decide that disclosure of confidential communication was required, but this should not be an easy and certainly not triumphant decision, but rather ultimately a failure of efforts to develop trust between doctor and patient.

It is clear that there are situations where the interest of society is compelling—morally compelling—and the professional may be obliged to abandon confidentiality. How should that decision be reached? Something within us would probably like a rule that might make such decisions easier, but there really is no such rule that would make decisions involving conflict of principles less anguishing.

I would suggest, however, that confidentiality is a principle that should be guarded by the careful vigilance of both the individual practitioner and social policy more generally. A society that does not respect confidentiality fails to protect the kind of privacy on which trust and intimate relationships are based. The consequences are chilling to imagine, not just for medicine but for the social fabric on which families, communities, and all intimate relationships depend.

CHAPTER 5

A CRITIQUE OF SZASZ'S CRITIQUE: THE MIND-BODY PROBLEM WON'T GO AWAY

THE LEGACY OF CARTESIAN DUALISM

The Cartesian approach to knowledge has greatly enhanced biomedical technology by liberating the study of man from medieval theology. Legitimizing the study of the human body as a thing, that is, as a physical entity (*res extensa*), has made possible great technical advances that could not have occurred if anatomical dissections and other experiments that might have challenged the authority of the church were prohibited. However, when we refer to the study of man in the traditions of philosophical anthropology, we understand that to mean much more than the study of human physiology. The "soul" (*res cogitans*), which Descartes split off from the body, has all but lost any compelling significance in modern culture; even the word "spirit" barely conveys the more-than-physical concerns that are inevitably a part of the physician's concern for the patient.

Thus our culture, for all its diversity, experiences the full force of the Cartesian legacy in modern medicine. It is now possible to conceive of medicine as an almost totally impersonal, technological enterprise, or it is possible to conceive of medicine in very personal terms and quite broadly as concerned with suffering of human beings. Medicine and physicians are criticized both for being too impersonal and for being concerned with too broad a range of problems. It is a paradox of our culture that medicine should be denounced for being too concerned with human suffering, while any number of purportedly radical critics of medicine—including Ralph Nader, Ivan Illych, and Thomas Szasz,[1] as well as members of the medical establishment—hold that medicine should limit its concern to strictly physical matters. It is also paradoxical that just as medical technology has really been able to demonstrate prodigious accomplishment, public satisfaction with medicine has been rapidly declining. The paradox here is not that the public is dissatisfied with medical technology, but that technical virtuosity has led the

71

physician to concentrate more on the physical aspects of disease with decreased concern for the patient who suffers. No one would wish a return to the turn-of-the-century physician, the "horse and buggy doctor," romantically remembered as sitting all night at the bedside of the dying patient, to whom he could offer little but compassion, but we might wish for more of the humane concern manifested by physicians of old.

It is one of the tasks of medical ethics to deal with this dichotomous view of medicine. Medical ethics is both the vehicle for transmitting professional tradition and the vehicle for calling those traditions into question. Recalling Chauncey Leake's distinction between matters of ethics and matters of etiquette, we may now paraphrase his concern as follows: While medical ethics is properly concerned with the ultimate conduct of physicians toward their patients and toward society as a whole, the consideration of the will and motive behind this conduct involves matters of etiquette and manners in medical practice. It is possible for ethics to avoid such personal, historical, and cultural considerations and to achieve explicit clarity on abstractly formulated questions, but it does so at the risk of further impersonalizing medical practice. Or to reformulate the problem: In order for medical ethics to achieve the kind of conceptual clarity that the Cartesian outlook requires, it must sacrifice any awareness of a whole, integrated, historical human being living in a cultural situation in favor of the Cartesian split personality. The Cartesian legacy in our culture leads us to *either* mentalistic *or* materialistic formulation of our problems, and this is especially the case in medicine.

Just as the appreciation of technology in our culture is ambivalent, so also is the appreciation of medicine. And herein lies the confusion, for medicine as an institution consists of individual physicians and patients, each unique by virtue of unique historical experiences, whatever experiences they may share as citizens of a particular culture. Physicians do not act in a cultural vacuum devoid of the expectations of their patients. Indeed for all the standardization of practices that medical technology has accomplished, the physician's practice starts with an assessment of the needs of each patient who appeals to the physician for help. It is often held that the so-called "medical model" entails certain values of a technological sort, namely, an approach to the body as thing as opposed to the patient as person, when in fact this may not be the case at all. What the medical model entails is ambiguous as is the scope of medical concern and the definitions of health and illness. The extremes may be distinguished by what Dr. Otto Guttentag calls "the biological medical model" and "the anthropological medical model" to avoid conceding that medicine is just concerned with physiological matters and, correspondingly, that doctors are unconcerned with people.[2]

Thus we see two basic ways in which Cartesian dualism can deter modern medicine: (1) through treating the body as a machine (*res extensa*) and (2) through the concept of discarnate mentality (*res cogitans*). The former is overly materialistic; the latter is overly rationalistic.[3] In all these chapters I have been discussing the limitations of an approach to ethics that attempts complete specifiability. In this chapter I attempt to demonstrate that this approach to ethics, depending as it does on an impersonal view of man (the person) and relying on the Cartesian mind-body dichotomy, contributes to the dehumanization experienced in modern medical practice.

THE DEFINITION OF MEDICINE

How is medicine to be conceived? What is the legitimate purview of the physician? Unquestionably the physician is to be concerned with physical illness: an infection, a myocardial infarction, a neoplasm. But what about "mental illness"? Should the physician be concerned with emotional problems, anxieties, depressions, psychoses? These concerns might once have been in the spiritual realm, the subject of religious counseling or advice. Does their legitimacy as medical problems stem from a demonstrated organic etiology, or do such mental problems stemming from "problems in living" legitimately belong in the medical purview? What about those patients who perceive themselves to have physical problems, but problems for which no organic etiology can be demonstrated? The polite term for them is "hypochondriacs"; they are sometimes disparagingly called "crocks" out of frustration; technically they are "conversion hysterics" if their symptom masquerade is unconscious, "malingerers" if it is conscious and willful. Should the physician be taking care of these people, or should they be refused admission to our hospitals and clinics? What about matters of preventive medicine, fluoridation, nutrition, sanitation, environmental pollution, industrial safety, family planning and birth control, abortion, nuclear energy and war, homosexuality, child abuse, and lifestyle including "bad habits" such as reckless driving, not using seatbelts, smoking, drinking, overeating, and underexercising? Should these matters be of no more concern to the physician than to any other citizen? Medicine is criticized for being both too much concerned and too little concerned with many of these areas.

There is no general agreement about these questions. There is a tradition of broad concern for the well-being of the patient that inclines the physician to adopt a broad definition of medicine. Notable in this tradition is Dr. Otto Guttentag, who defines medicine as "the care of health of human beings by human beings" to stress the physician's fellow-concern for another human being.[4] Also in this tradition is the World Health Organization definition of medicine, which stresses physical, emotional, and social well-being. Yet there is another tradition that says the physician should tend only to matters of physical disease. Many of today's young physicians and medical students are defensively adopting this posture in response to the more hostile of medicine's critics. "Why take unnecessary risks, which aren't appreciated anyway? Better to specialize narrowly in an area where I can be sure of my competence," they are saying. Others, sensing a growing resentment of medical paternalism, will say, equally defensively, "Patients are responsible for their health; if they want to kill themselves by smoking, I can't stop them. I will help those who ask for my help."

These are issues that no physician escapes. Whether or not they are presented in an ethical context, they are dealt with as physicians make choices about how they will practice medicine, as well as how they will handle each encounter with each patient. Inevitably there are differences in expectations in any human encounter, no less so in the doctor-patient encounter. Often patients will come to physicians expecting something other than what the physician is prepared to offer. Undoubtedly clarification of expectations should be very much part of the negotiations between physician and patient and involve them together in planning a treatment upon which both agree. A frequent problem is that physicians do not adequately ask patients to clarify their expectations or do not adequately explain the treatments they recommend, just as it is a problem that patients are often surreptitious about stating what they want. A patient may complain of back pain, for example, leading the physician to believe that the patient wishes to be relieved of the symptoms when in fact they are tolerable, and the patient's conscious desire is that the physician aid in gaining monetary compensation in a legal dispute; unconsciously the patient may want dependency gratification, but not cure.

One way of clarifying these differing expectations is to distinguish between disease and illness. Though disease and illness are practically synonymous in everyday usage, they are not necessarily the same thing, and herein lies the confusion. *Illnesses* are experiences of disvalued changes in states of being and in social function; *diseases*, in the scientific paradigm of modern medicine, are abnormalities in the structure and function of body organs and systems. To state the distinction tersely: Patients suffer illnesses; physicians (in the Cartesian paradigms, which reduce life to physics and chemistry) diagnose and treat diseases.[5]

Disease and illness may not always occur simultaneously. A patient may complain of symptoms for which the doctor can find no organic explanation, or conversely the doctor may make a diagnosis of disease that the patient does not experience as illness. In the former category are conversion hysteria and malingering; in the latter are hypertension and asymptomatic diabetes, which may subsequently become illnesses if the patient does not comply with the doctor's prescriptions. The following chart (Figure 5) illustrates some of the dichotomous possibilities and the value choices that must be made by both physicians and patients in determining the role of medicine in their lives.

Just as the perception of a problem as an illness or a disease may change from time to time in any given individual, so also may the perception in a society change. Masturbation, for example, was widely considered an illness around the turn of the century. Now, with recognition of its statistical "normality," it is no longer considered a medical problem, even though many people

74

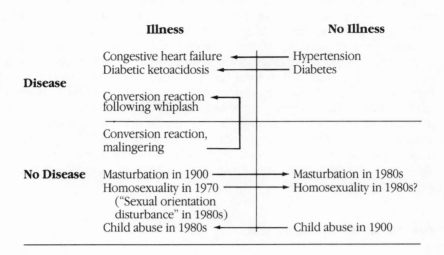

still experience feelings of shame and guilt about masturbation, perhaps not so much about the act itself as about the fantasies that accompany masturbation.[6] Many forms of behavior that were once considered moral problems or "perversions" have been humanistically appropriated into the medical realm, relabeled as illness or perhaps even as diseases, and given the supposedly value-neutral status of "deviations." Alcoholism and sexual perversions might fit in this category. Homosexuality was formally reclassified in 1974 by the American Psychiatric Association and removed from the *Diagnostic and Statistical Manual of Mental Disorders Second Edition,* being replaced by "Sexual Orientation Disturbance (Homosexuality)." This move presumably was made because not all people who claimed the identity of homosexuality considered themselves to be ill. Thus what was recently a moral problem, a "perversion," was demoralized and medicalized as a "deviation" and then partially demedicalized as an "elective form of sexual behavior." The process works the other way too, as exemplified by the situation of child abuse, which is now viewed as a medical problem. This change reflects in part the new ability of psychotherapists and community agencies to identify the problem and then intervene and offer "treatment."

Value choices reflecting cultural attitudes are made at a most fundamental level concerning "sickness" (disease and/or illness). Not only in the examples discussed to illustrate the scope of possibilities, but in any number of situations that come to the physician's attention, decisions must be made as to what should be the physician's best response to the request for help. Often in our culture the problem is perceived to be *either* a physical *or* a mental problem, the latter being the province of the psychiatrist as the specialists who deals with functional or nonorganic problems. Thus there is confusion about the relationship of mind to body. This can be understood by considering the relationship of psychiatry to the rest of medicine. Cartesian dualism creates something of an identity problem for psychiatry, depending on how one perceives the medical model. Some adherents of "biological psychiatry" hold that psychiatry's legitimate place in medicine is derived from its treatment of mental problems with a biological basis, "biological" being understood to mean "physical-chemical." This view accepts the supremacy of the biological medical model. Alternatively, others such as George Engel argue that the medical model must be understood to encompass not only biological phenomenon but bio-psychosocial problems, broadly conceived.[7] The dichotomy itself is spurious, but focusing on it provides a useful context for understanding some of the debates in medical ethics, which take the Cartesian epistemological outlook for granted.

THE "MYTH" OF MENTAL ILLNESS

Questions of ethics lead to questions of philosophical anthropology: How is a human being to be conceived of in medicine? Since Cartesianism splits man into mind and body, conceived dichotomously, we have been led to consider the place of psychiatry in medicine and in relation to the rest of medicine. The physician is often presented with the question as to whether a certain problem is physical or emotional, "mental" or some variant of a nonphysical problem. Faced with such dichotomous alternatives, we may say medicine should be limited to the strictly physical, or we may say that medicine should be broadly defined to include mental or emotional problems. I have been arguing for the more-encompassing and personal approach. Thomas Szasz takes exactly the opposite approach: He argues that medicine's only proper concern is physical illness and that mental illness is a myth.

Szasz is aware of the impact of Cartesianism on medicine and accepts it as proper and inevitable. Without imagining alternatives, Szasz does not face the question of how to conceive of medicine; but rather in accepting the Cartesian dichotomy, he faces the questions of how to conceive of moral problems, problems in living, and problems involving human ambiguity in a system that insists on conceptual clarity. Says Szasz, "Strictly speaking, disease or illness can affect only the body; hence, there can be no mental illness."[8]

Since we are prepared to consider alternatives to the Cartesian system, which Szasz is not, we must consider the full import of Szasz's statement for our conception of medicine. "Myth" itself has many possible interpretations. In the Cartesian system and as Szasz uses it, "myth" refers to a nonreality, something that is not to be believed. Alternatively, to a cultural anthropologist or to a theologian a myth is a system of belief, which organizes the way reality is to be understood in a particular culture or religion. Thus we may understand the myth of mental illness to mean a nonreality in which we should not

76

believe or a reflection of the organizing beliefs of our culture, a way of understanding reality. As Polanyi points out, "if we equate the real with the tangible, then minds may not seem real, even though they are in a sense more real than stones, which are tangible." Similarly if we expect illnesses to be tangible in order to be real, then we may easily conclude that mental illnesses are not real, though they are real indeed to those who suffer from them.

Szasz rightly deserves to be criticized for his overreliance on the Cartesian outlook, his overly narrow conception of medicine, and most especially for his absolute opposition to involuntary commitment of mental patients. But I cite his work not just to discredit it, for he is among the most prominent contributors to medical and psychiatric ethics, discussing many issues with a nuance of understanding and a sensitivity that is uncommon. Rather I cite Szasz to demonstrate how, even with the kind of sensitivity he shows, it is possible to come to some very rigid conclusions that may actually make matters worse rather than better—and do so in the name of ethics.

UNDERSTANDING HYSTERIA

Particularly to Szasz's credit and indispensable for our understanding of contemporary medicine's dilemmas is his analysis of hysteria, which he uses as a prototype of the myth of mental illness, but which we might use equally well as a basis for understanding medicine in personal rather than physical terms. He cites Freud's account of Charcot's pioneering work on hysteria:

> [Charcot] explained that the theory of organic nervous diseases was for the present fairly complete, and he began to turn his attention almost exclusively to hysteria, thus suddenly focusing general attention to this subject. This most enigmatic of all nervous diseases—no workable point of view having yet been found from which physicians could regard it—had just at this time come very much into discredit. . . . First of all Charcot's work restored dignity to the subject; gradually the sneering attitude, which the hysteric could reckon on meeting when she told her story, was given up; she was no longer a malingerer, since Charcot had thrown the whole weight of his authority on the side of the reality and objectivity of the hysterical phenomenon.[9]

Thus by virtue of his authority, according to this account, Charcot restored a modicum of human dignity to those who suffered from nonorganic illness. It remained for Freud himself, initially in collaboration with Breuer, to further dignify the illness by explaining how and why the hysteric suffered and by offering a method for treating the hysteric's symptoms. Breuer discovered that the symptoms disappeared if the patient recalled under hypnosis the time when the symptoms first appeared. Freud later found that hypnosis was unnecessary and substituted the method of free association, by which analyst and patient working together could come to understand the origin and meaning of the symptoms and possibly find alternative ways of dealing with heretofore unconscious conflict.

77

Observing these historical "facts," a value judgment must be made. Was what Freud did good or was it bad? Szasz makes an interesting observation in this regard. He notes that,

> Although Freud regarded hysteria as a disease, he clearly understood it far better than his language allowed him to express it. He was in a sort of semantic and epistemological straitjacket from which he freed himself only rarely and for brief periods. The following passage is an example of description in plain language, unencumbered by the need to impress the reader that the "patient" is truly ill and a genuine patient.[10]

Szasz then goes on to quote Freud's account:

> Here, then, was the unhappy story of this proud girl with her longing for love. Unreconciled to her fate, embittered by the failure of all her little schemes for reestablishing the family's former glories, with those she loved dead or gone away or estranged, unready to take refuge in the love of some unknown man—she had lived for eighteen months in almost complete seclusion, with nothing to occupy her but the care of her mother and her own pains.[11]

Szasz is entirely correct that Freud relied heavily on scientific or mechanistic paradigms in explaining his theories, perhaps in order to make them intelligible to the scientific community. He used those paradigms metaphorically to explain the suffering of hysterical persons (usually women) who presented themselves to physicians (originally neurologists, then psychiatrists) asking for help. Freud was thoroughly scientific insofar as he relied closely on his observations to draw his conclusions, but not in his reliance on mechanical terminology to explain emotional and moral phenomena. Use of such terms as "forces," "determinants," "impulses" and the like have left Freud open to the criticism that he was "reductionistic," though it should be acknowledged that he wisely decided not to publish "Project for a Scientific Psychology" (1895), where he speculates on the physiological determinants of behavior.[12] Thus a critic such as Szasz might well go on to reinterpret the moral dimension of the suffering hysteric, but instead he himself remains locked in the same Cartesian straitjacket that he claimed was shackling Freud. Szasz, faced with the same moral dilemma that Freud faced and faced with the same "facts," arrives at a different value judgment; namely, that it is not the physician's place to help these people because they do not suffer from "real" illnesses.

INVOLUNTARY HOSPITALIZATION

It could be argued that it matters little whether mental illness is considered a myth or a reality as long as one is sensitive to the value dimensions involved in making such a choice and as long as the value judgments are acknowledged as such. Both Freud and Szasz are exquisitely sensitive to such issues. But there is one problem that cannot be overlooked in this analysis and that is the possibility of moral inversion when moral ideals are held as absolute moral imperatives. I believe Szasz falls prey to this problem in his conclusion that involuntary commitment should be absolutely prohibited on the grounds that there is no such thing as mental illness. Consider the following example:

> *A 23-year-old mother was transferred from the obstetrics service to the psychiatry ward because of disturbing fantasies that she might harm her baby by stuffing rags into its mouth. Three days later she was released against medical advice when she insisted she had to take care of her baby. Two days after that she returned to the Emergency Room saying that she could not tolerate her baby and was afraid she might hurt it. She refused admission but was committed.*
>
> *A team of civil liberties lawyers opposed the commitment and opposed efforts of the Social Services agency to take legal custody of the baby. They argued that she had a "right" to care for her baby, and that attempts to separate her from the baby would only make her worse. After several months involving several court appearances, she was arrested for creating a public disturbance. In jail she hanged herself, not deprived of her civil rights, but deprived of the psychiatric help she so desperately needed.*

The dilemmas posed by this patient are illustrative of the kinds of concerns that must be dealt with, but that an absolutist approach fails to adequately consider. We see a very real conflict between opposing moral principles with a beneficent treatment offered in the patient's best interest on one hand and the abstract principle of liberty on the other, even though that may not be in the patient's best interest. Any action in such a situation will be less than perfect because conflicting ideals are involved. Were the patient perfectly rational, there would be no problem, but she says at one minute that she wants to be in the hospital; the next minute she does not. Her psychopathology does not allow her to integrate her impulses over time. It is the very ambiguity of the situation that the civil liberties lawyers (and Szasz), expecting matters to be clear and distinct in strict Cartesian fashion, cannot tolerate. To clarify such ambiguity and to defend against the dreadful anxiety of trying to empathize with the schizophrenic turmoil, the civil liberties lawyer abstracts certain facts from the complexity and tenaciously insists on nothing less than moral perfection, which is determined a priori with no reference to the needs of the individual patient.

This may be considered moral inversion because the moral thing to do would be to provide this confused woman with a stable environment where her impulses could be controlled and integrated over time; that is, to insure psychiatric care for her, or, to translate this concern into the language of rights, to insure her right to treatment. What the schizophrenic woman needs is not an adversarial proceeding designed to obtain an abstract clarity at her expense, but rather a cooperative exploration of how her needs can best be met with all interested parties attempting to formulate a plan that guarantees her right to the best treatment available without violating her civil rights. Such an approach, admittedly novel in our judicial system, would properly be called fiduciary insofar as it would rest on trust and cooperation, rather than control and competition, between parties with different methods and outlooks but with similar goals, namely, the interests of the patient.

An exhaustive analysis of all the legal, medical, and moral aspects of the issue of involuntary commitment is beyond the scope of this inquiry. My purpose in raising the issue in this context is to relocate the issue that I believe cannot be ignored—the conception of the person. A view that focuses on "freedom" as an absolute or on civil liberties, however desirable, without also accounting for the attendant limitations, such as the limitation of the mental patient to think rationally, is inevitably incomplete.[13] What it means to think rationally is something which, of course, must be interpreted epistemologically, and that is where the debate should be located. In the chapter on informed consent it is possible to say more about how these judgments might responsibly be made.

THE ETHICS OF GIVING PLACEBOS

The person suffering from nonorganic "ills" is not always identified as a psychiatric patient. Many people come to the doctor with poorly defined symptoms, experienced perhaps as pains in the body. In areas where it may be possible to obtain psychiatric consultation, these problems may be translated into psychiatric problems and a treatment approach developed that attempts to get at the etiology of the problem. But in many instances the problems may be treated symptomatically, perhaps with a placebo medication. The patient may benefit also from the placebo effect of the encounter with the physician, someone who listens to the patient, does not criticize or demean, and "seems to understand."

Into these therapeutic encounters enter matters of clinical judgment for the physician, value judgments that can and should be subject to ethical reflection. As with so many ethical issues, care must be taken in asking the proper questions and keeping a clear distinction between matters of value and interpretations of fact. On the specific matter of placebos, for example, do we raise the issue as a matter of "truth-telling" or do we inquire into the best method for caring for the hysterical patient in a medical system that reflects a culture tending to maintain rather sharp divisions between problems of the mind and problems of the body?

Sissela Bok analyzes placebos as an issue of truth-telling, actually as an example of lying. Her analysis is informative not only on the use of placebos, but also on the pitfalls of ethical analysis based on the Cartesian assumption of a mind-body split. Bok quite correctly realizes that lying exacts a toll, namely an erosion of trust, as much for the liar as for the victim of the deception. But in her fervor to denounce lying, she overlooks the importance of a careful search to understand the truth.

> Applied ethics, then, has seemed uncongenial and lacking in theoretical chal-
> lenge to many moral philosophers even apart from any belief in epistemological
> priority and from muddles about the meaning of "truth." As a result, practical
> moral choice comes to be given short shrift, and never more so than in the case
> of lies.[14]

Her point is an important one, and her assessment that many epistemological discussions lead to "muddles" about what the truth is should serve as a
warning to fellow philosophers not to ignore urgent practical problems in
favor of theoretical issues. Nonetheless, the theoretical questions remain, and
an understanding of what the truth is remains indispensable to any decision
about when, if ever, it might be acceptable to lie. Bok's arguments about lying
are essentially valid, but she has difficulty applying them to the practical
situation of deciding whether to give placebos because she does not adequately settle the antecedent questions. She recognizes that the prevailing
outlook is inadequate but immediately falls prey to its seductive familiarity.

Bok is a victim of our culture. Without awareness of accounts of knowledge alternative to the Cartesian demand for explicitness, she understandably
misperceives an epistemological issue as an ethical problem, as we are all
inclined to do. When asked how we like the new necktie Uncle Joe sent, for
example, we often understand the request as requiring an (objective) assessment about the tie, rather than an invitation to say something about ourselves,
our (aesthetic) values, our tastes, and our judgments. We lie and say the tie is
lovely (a white lie, to be sure; maybe trivial), when in fact once again we so
easily substitute a statement of fact for the disclosure of a judgment of value.

Ethically, a question even more difficult than whether to lie is how to
understand and communicate the truth: how to understand what Uncle Joe
really wants to know and how to tell him our feelings, not only about the tie
but about himself. For the physician the question is how to understand the
patient's human as well as physical needs and how best to serve those needs.
To decide when and how to tell a patient he has cancer, the oncologist must
understand more than cancer; he must know the patient as well.

THE DIFFERENCE BETWEEN PLACEBOS AND THE PLACEBO EFFECT

Locked in the grip of Cartesian dualism, it seems only natural to consider the
placebo a lie. It does not cause a direct physiological intervention in the *body*.
It does something to the *mind* instead. This is problematic if one conceives of
medicine as a technology intended to intervene in the body's mechanisms
rather than a service profession intended to help people.

Medicine's identity as a profession fringes on our understanding of personhood. Is a person something more than a mind in a machine? Do we perceive ourselves as having any psychosomatic integrity, or are our bodies alien to ourselves? William Poteat in a startling new work, *Polanyian Meditations*, coins a new conjoined word, "mindbody," to remind us how habitual the Cartesian split has become in our way of thinking about ourselves.[15] The language of (w)holism might be useful here as a way of getting beyond the mind-body dualism. Certainly treating the whole person is a legitimate aim of medicine. Yet the concept of "wholistic medicine," however noble its aims, is often used as a reaction to mechanistic medicine and produces a reductionistic spiritualism or "psychism" that is every bit as one-sided as the poison to which it is supposed to be the antidote.

The problems Bok attempts to deal with as ethical questions recur as matters of genuine perplexity for physicians in clinical practice. Those patients for whom placebos may legitimately be a more ethical option than using dangerously addicting analgesics may be called "hysterics" or "placebo-responders," but they must be recognized as fellow human beings in need of help and cannot be dismissed as moral degenerates by the physician, the medical profession, or critics of the medical profession, no matter how frustrating, time-consuming, or expensive their care may be. The mind-body problem recurs as the basis of so many problems in medical ethics and the practice of medicine in part because hysterics refuse to think of themselves and refuse to experience their bodies in the ways demanded by Cartesian notions of rationality. One of the differences between practicing medicine and reflecting on the practice of medicine is that the physician must actually deal with (often irrational) fellow human beings and not just idealized approximations thereof. The doctor-patient relationship, therefore, continues to be an important focus for understanding ethical dilemmas that issue from medical practice.

CHAPTER 6

INFORMED CONSENT, AUTONOMY, AND PATERNALISM: RESPECTING THE PATIENT IN RESEARCH AND PRACTICE

INFORMED CONSENT has evolved into a central position in ethical thinking about the relationship between psychiatrists and their patients, especially in research settings. Redlich and Mollica state that "informed consent is the basis of all psychiatric intervention and that without it no psychiatric intervention can be morally justified. The only exception would be a patient judged incompetent to give his informed consent, preferably by a court."[1] Yet the notion of informed consent is caught between two divergent approaches to ethics, which leave much ambiguity as to how the concept of informed consent should be applied to psychiatric patients. One approach argues that the requirement is based on the principle of autonomy and that we require informed consent because persons have a right to self-determination. This view is problematic with psychiatric patients and other groups considered "nonautonomous," such as children, prisoners, the senile, the comatose, and participants in research involving deception, all of whom may lack the inner freedom to exercise a truly informed consent.

The other approach rests on the benevolent concern for fellow human beings, which may require a "paternalistic" judgment about what may be in the best interest of a particular patient. Some critics have suggested that the protectionist stance of informed consent is intended to protect a presumably helpless person from the inequities of power that may occur in relationships with professionals.[2-7] Psychiatrists are often cast in the defensive position of being unduly paternalistic or of being insufficiently concerned with the rights of their patients. On the contrary, however, a psychodynamic understanding of the nature of dependency relationships and of the development of independence broadens the understanding of autonomy beyond the ways in which it is usually applied to questions of informed consent and offers an alternative to the objectionable idea that psychiatric patients and others considered nonautonomous are somehow a different category of persons.

Furthermore, the psychodynamic approach suggests a model for informed consent generally.

If we think about informed consent as an action of the autonomous person, we are left at an impasse about how to treat the nonautonomous person. The nonautonomous person is not necessarily to be excluded from participation in psychiatric research or procedures. But we must carefully consider how best to protect both the rights and interests of those whose capabilities are limited. To state my argument as succinctly as possible: I believe that our Western intellectual traditions have led us dangerously close to equating personhood with rationality and that overly legalistic notions of informed consent actually work to the detriment of persons with diminished capabilities—and to the detriment of all of us—by emphasizing criteria that divide us from one another. After sketching the contours of the problem, I will propose a way of thinking about informed consent that relies more on the relationships between people than it does on the notion of an isolated and autonomous person.

THE PRINCIPLE OF AUTONOMY

Current legal and philosophical justification for informed consent rests on the principle of autonomy.[8] The principle of autonomy holds that individuals are the possessors of individual rights, including the right to self-determination. Far from being an unassailable doctrine, the notion of autonomy is subject to internal contradiction. It is linked to notions of personal freedom, which do not adequately account for how that freedom is to be achieved. Kant stressed freedom of the will in contrasting autonomy with heteronomy (rule by external sources, other persons or conditions). Autonomy for Kant meant governing oneself in accord with moral principles that are one's own and that could be willed to be universally valid. John Stuart Mill stressed autonomy of action in which the autonomous individual is free from social control. In both the deontological tradition of Kant and the utilitarian tradition of Mill, which have so largely shaped modern ethical theory, autonomy is seen as an achievement of rational cognition with little understanding of how that cognition is acquired or of the limitations of such autonomy. Autonomy is not merely a cognitive achievement, but involves the whole person, including his or her affective states and developmental history. The elucidation of how autonomy emerges from dependency and social relationships in families and communities, not from isolated cognition, has come largely from psychiatric and psychoanalytic thinking. Erikson, for example, discusses autonomy as a developmental stage occurring around the time when the child is beginning to gain mastery over musculature for locomotion and sphincter control.[9] The achievement of autonomy serves as a defense against feelings of shame and doubt, but the failure to achieve autonomy leaves one dependent or seeking dependency throughout life. Margaret Mahler describes the tasks of this stage of development as separation-individuation, a process that begins with loco-motion but which may never be completed in some individuals.[10] Autonomy has its origins in a state of dependency. It is a task of development, a goal to be achieved rather than a moral absolute.

The principle of autonomy has the merit of bolstering the individual against possible violations of trust. It has the liability of degenerating to an abstraction, of being applied to persons in isolation, or of being applied to groups without due regard for the idiosyncrasies of individuals. Though there is widespread acceptance of the idea that the principle of autonomy is indeed the basis of our requirement for informed consent, I am concerned that our preoccupation with autonomy as an absolute has become an obsession reaching pathological proportions, allowing us to distance ourselves bureau-cratically from those who suffer and from the painful realities of being sick, dependent, and in need of help.

THE ASSESSMENT OF COMPETENCE

If we rely on the principle of autonomy as the basis for our requirement of informed consent, we are faced with problems about what to do with those persons who cannot be said to be autonomous. By a strictly legal interpreta-tion of informed consent, the right to self-determination cannot be exercised without the ability to understand the information. This creates a conflict with the exercise of another right, the right to participate in procedures or research that may be of benefit to oneself or others. This conflict is usually resolved, not by questioning the concept of autonomy, but by declaring the nonautonomous person as also not competent.

A person's competence may vary from situation to situation or from time to time. A person may be competent to make certain decisions but not others. As Beauchamp and Childress have observed,

> The notions of limited competence and intermittent competence are useful, because they require a statement of the precise decisions a person can make, while avoiding the false dichotomy of "either competent or incompetent." Use of these notions preserves maximum autonomy, justifying intervention only in those instances where a person clearly is of questionable competence.[11]

Competency is a legal concept and all individuals are presumed by law to be competent until determined otherwise by a judicial hearing. The practical realities of clinical care often require an assessment of competence to refuse or consent to a particular procedure. Appelbaum and Roth[12] stress the dy-namic qualities of competence for which static legal theories do not make adequate provision. They draw a distinction between "psychological capacity" and "legal competence." They suggest five criteria that should be used in assessing competency: (1) psychodynamic elements of the patient's personality; (2) the accuracy of the historical information conveyed by the patient; (3) the accuracy and completeness of the information disclosed to the patient; (4) the stability of the patient's mental status over time; and (5) the effect of the setting in which consent is obtained.[12] These criteria help broaden the concept of competence to be responsive to the needs of a particular person at a particular time.

Stanley and Stanley have detailed some of the negative consequences of a protective attitude toward the mentally ill regarding informed consent. They note that the mentally ill are often grouped together with regard to needing special protection. It is assumed that their judgment and thinking are impaired in a manner that makes them unable to make independent judgments. It is also reasoned that their illness leaves them vulnerable to exploitation. Special protection for such patients is designed to prevent such exploitation. Yet the inadvertent negative consequences of such protectionism need to be considered.[13]

One major negative effect of a protective stance toward the mentally ill, the Stanleys note, is paradoxically a loss of autonomy. Decisions as to whether to select a certain treatment or participate in certain research are taken at least partially out of their hands. Thus their right to decide their own fate is viewed as secondary to assuring that they are not exploited. Furthermore, the mentally ill are defined and labeled as different from others, specifically more vulnerable and less capable of evaluating situations with regard to their self-interest. This arbitrary grouping of a highly heterogeneous population may inadvertently give tacit societal approval for discrimination against this group. In an effort to protect them, another stigma is added to being classified as mentally ill. The implication of requiring special protection is that psychiatric patients are incapable of functioning as autonomous persons.

Finally, protective policies may have the inadvertent effect of infantilizing patients by removing some of their decision-making power. The message given to the patients is that their judgment is poor and they need to be cared for. This may ultimately contribute to the lowering of self-esteem in the mentally ill and a fostering of unnecessary dependency. Protectiveness is a double-edged sword. While it must be recognized that good reasons exist for safeguards in that abuses can and have occurred, the therapeutic goals of increased patient autonomy, which most would recognize, must be kept in mind in applying the safeguards, lest protectiveness work against the best interests of the patient.

TOWARD A DEFINITION OF INFORMED CONSENT

Strictly speaking, informed consent has three components: It must be (1) informed, (2) voluntary, and (3) competent. Consent should include such elements as the following: (1) a fair explanation of the procedures or treatments, (2) a description of discomforts and risks, (3) a description of expected benefits, (4) disclosure of alternate procedures, (5) an offer to answer any inquiries, (6) an instruction that the person is free to withdraw consent and discontinue participation in the project or activity, and (7) a statement that withdrawal will not result in a loss of benefits or prejudice treatment. These are but minimal standards. It cannot be assumed that once these requirements are met the physician or investigator has no further obligations to the patient or experimental subject.

"Consent" in the dictionary definition is derived from the Latin *com-* plus *sentire*; to feel, hence to feel together. It means "agree," "assent," or "give permission" and indicates involvement of the will or feelings and compliance with what is requested or desired. Implicit in the definition of consent is a community of feeling, a shared trust. With recognition of this mutuality, Guttentag offers a useful definition of informed consent:

> Informed consent may be defined as the experimenter's willing obligation to inform the experimental subject, to the best of the experimenter's knowledge, about the personal risk that the experimental subject faces in the proposed experiment, the significance of the experiment for the advancement of knowledge and human welfare, and last but not least, the stakes involved for the experimenter himself. In short, informed consent implies that the experimenter has made the most honest effort he can to say everything that will enhance the experimental subject's freedom, so that the subject can make the most adequate choice of which he is capable in agreeing or refusing to become a volunteer.[14]

THE PRINCIPLE OF PARTNERSHIP

More basic than the principle of autonomy is the principle of partnership, which stems not from the fact that certain persons are different from ourselves, but rather from the commonness we share with our fellow human beings. In a highly personal approach to ethics, Guttentag offers the notion of "partnership" as the basic principle in experiments involving human subjects:

> With reference to the relationship between experimenter and experimental subject, it is the concept of partnership between the two, resulting from the fact of their being fellow human beings, that reflects our basic belief and cannot be subordinated to any other.[15]

By partnership Guttentag does not imply a legal contract or business association, but "sincerity without reserve, a relationship of mutual trust and confidence, or openness between experimenter and subject, and a blind reliance that discards any guardedness." A criterion of this partnership, Guttentag insists, is the personal effort involved in its enactment, "the amount of 'loving care,' or devotion given to disclosing to the experimental subject and to 'mankind' the content and limits of any actual partnership. It is the antipode to negligence."

Reliance on the notion of partnership may serve as a reminder that important personal elements are involved in the maintenance of the highest ethical standards. Furthermore, such words as "trust," "sincerity," and "loving care" serve to stress a dimension of ethical responsibility that is omitted in the modern ethical vocabulary of minimalist operational guidelines.

It is this principle of partnership that represents the ideal of the physician's ethic even more fundamentally than the beneficent paternalism of which medicine is often accused or than the more remote concept of autonomy, which is often substituted. The work of the psychiatrist in psychotherapy offers a prototype of the working partnership. In psychotherapy the establishment of a trusting alliance is one of the first tasks in therapy, one which is a prerequisite for all the work that follows. The working alliance of the psychoanalyst and the neurotic analysand offers a model for understanding informed consent in any context. Here the "experimenter" and "experimental subject/patient" have one overriding goal in their joint work together and that is to understand as much as possible about the motives of the life of the latter. The ambiguities of communication are taken with utmost seriousness and respect. The overdetermined as well as self-determined qualities of human action are appreciated in each step of self-understanding. The psychotherapeutic partners recognize that an articulated statement may have many levels of meaning, conscious and unconscious, and that not all can be appreciated simultaneously. Informed consent in the psychotherapeutic experiment occurs not once but continually, as the partners work together to bring into conscious awareness that which had hitherto been unknown.

The transaction of an informed consent inevitably relies on the use of language, which is meant to clarify but which might also confuse or conceal. Unless one assumes that an articulated statement can be understood literally, it is always a challenging task to discern meaning in what people say. This is especially the case with psychiatric patients. When a hospitalized patient announces that he wishes to be discharged immediately to attend to important business matters, he may be responding to mundane necessity or he may be manifesting psychotic grandiosity. His statement of intent may be a veiled test of his physician—"Do you really care about me?"—or it may be a realistic protest against his incarceration. If his condition were serious enough to warrant treatment with electroconvulsive therapy, could his consent for the procedure be considered valid? Conversely, in face of a potentially life-threatening situation such as starvation due to catatonic schizophrenia or catatonic depression, would an articulated refusal be grounds for not treating the condition?

An example from clinical experience illustrates the difficulties of attending to the meaning in articulated statements, when such statements contain manifest ambivalence:

Mrs. J. was admitted to the plastic surgery service of a teaching hospital for skin grafts on an ulcerated foot. She was transferred to the psychiatry service when she became disoriented and disruptive. She was brought to a teaching conference for a diagnostic interview. A medical student was designated to interview Mrs. J. The interview went something as follows:

Medical student: *Good morning, Mrs. J., Could you tell us something about how you came to be here and how we might be of help to you?*
Mrs. J.: *I don't want to be here and I don't want to answer any questions.*
Medical student: *How long have you been in the hospital?*
Mrs. J.: *Don't talk to me.*
Medical student: *Have you been told why you are on the psychiatry service?*
Mrs. J.: *How would you feel if someone made you come to this conference?*
Medical student: *I think I know how you feel. (Pause) Are you married?*
Mrs. J.: *(Angrily) Don't you think that's a little bit personal, Sonny?*
Medical student: *Would you rather not answer that question?*
Mrs. J.: *I've been married twice and divorced twice.*

From that point on, the interview proceeded relatively smoothly with Mrs. J. disclosing relevant aspects of her life history and current situation. After the interview was concluded, another medical student inquired if informed consent had been obtained for the interview. Although hospital rules do not require a formal informed consent for an interview, the question was germane, especially in view of Mrs. J.'s articulated statement that she did not wish to be interviewed. However, when offered the option of not answering the question, she chose to answer in personal detail. At the very least we could say that Mrs. J. was ambivalent about the interview and that there was more to her feelings than her articulated statement indicated. The medical student, by respecting her wish for distance and control and by not responding defensively or punitively to the negative side of her ambivalence, was able to establish himself as someone worthy of Mrs. J.'s trust. As Mrs. J. became less antagonistic, she was able to acknowledge her fears without becoming overwhelmed by them. Although there is no correct solution to the medical student's dilemma, the interview could have been terminated for lack of adequately informed consent, thereby protecting the patient's right of refusal but ignoring the possibility of helping her.

BEYOND THE IMPASSE

The act of obtaining an informed consent involves us in two contradictory activities simultaneously. On the one hand, we strive for conceptual clarity in a full disclosure of the information. On the other hand, we abandon such abstract clarity on behalf of the person who must understand the consent form. One effort stresses the information in the consent form. The other effort stresses the process of consenting. This process relies heavily on the ethical integrity of the clinician or investigator not to violate the trust of the patient/ subject.

Solutions to this dilemma that focus on the information aspect of informed consent are inadequate. Examining the subjects on the contents of the form would disclose more about test-taking skills than the subjects' intentions. A categorical exclusion of psychiatric patients or subjects with diminished competence would insure against violations in the process of informed consent, but in itself risks violating certain rights such as the right to participate in the search for knowledge about one's own illness. The traditional "proxy consent" substitutes another person for the experimental subject, a person who presumably is more capable of understanding the information in the consent form but who may or may not be in a good position to speak for the interests of the patient/subject.

The requirement of the physician to maintain trust and good faith in negotiating the informed consent is a standard too high to be regulated. Traditionally the relationship between doctor and patient is spoken of as a fiduciary relationship, a relationship based on mutual trust. For the physician, the minimal limits of regulatory guidelines are necessary and useful but not ethically sufficient. The physician must be open to the greater trust placed in him or her by the patient. Even if the investigator as a person maintains the highest ethical standards, there is a potential conflict of interest because of the investigator's parallel commitment to the outcome of the investigation. Since the physician-scientist has a conflicting loyalty to the patient and to the outcome of the investigation, the trust of the physician-scientist cannot be assumed. It has been suggested that it may then be necessary to separate the roles of the physician-friend and the physician-scientist.[16, 17]

If keep in mind the simultaneous movements in obtaining an informed consent, the basis for separation becomes evident. We have:

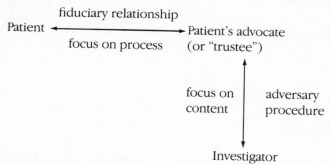

While the ethical physician or investigator should be able to keep such conflicts of interest in focus, it is important to be aware of the moral ambiguity intrinsic in such relationships. This moral ambiguity and the problems of protective paternalism do not go away by involving a third person in the decision-making process. The delineation of separate roles, however, serves as a useful ethical reminder to those who ask others to make informed choices about research or treatment in which they themselves have a stake.

Recognition of the dimension of time in the decision-making process resolves the contradiction posed by the rival ethical theories for the problem of informed consent. The juxtaposition of autonomy and paternalism, seen as mutually exclusive attitudes in medical practice and research, is unfortunate and misleading. Whereas paternalism might once have been seen as a manifestation of the physician's responsibility, it is now largely seen as a measure of the professional's control over the patient. The paternalistic physician is seen as limiting patient autonomy; the autonomous patient is seen as not needing to be dependent on the physician. What is missing from this analysis is the dimension of time. The statistic formulations of the physician as paternalistic or of the patient as autonomous are characterizations that may approximate a given person at a particular instant, but say nothing about their relationship over time.

Viewing informed consent as an ongoing process in a fiduciary relationship reestablishes the higher ethical sense of responsibility. The physician's (or investigator's) responsibility is a response to the needs of the patient/subject. Informed consent in such a model is not performed once but over and over again throughout the duration of the relationship. Appelbaum and Roth have suggested that an education model might be a more appropriate conceptualization of what is sought in informed consent.[18] Recognizing the dependency that may occur in such relationships, it might be appropriate to view informed consent in legitimately paternalistic (or at least parental) terms. The concern for the patient/subject is like that of a responsible parent for his or her child: Autonomy is seen as a desirable goal toward which they both work, but it is not taken as a given. Only in indifference does one treat a child or a patient or a research subject as completely autonomous. Autonomy is the goal of a therapeutic relationship; it is not the basis for our ethical concern for our fellow human beings.

INFORMED CONSENT IN GREAT BRITAIN

We have become so accustomed in the United States to the consumerist notions of autonomy and we accord so much respect to the standards of informed consent enshrined in the Declaration of Geneva that it may be worth looking at the issue in cross-cultural perspective. The issues of freedom and human rights by which we customarily orient ourselves in "Western civilization" are by no means universal and even in Western countries are understood differently.

The application of informed consent to treatment has been given increasing attention in the legal and ethical literature of the past two decades, resulting in "liberation" of the mental health laws of most Western countries.[19]

Legislation usually entails some form of due process review for involuntary psychiatric hospitalization and may also specify review for other procedures. An example of the latter is the stipulation in Great Britain's Mental Health Act 1983, which requires that consent *and* a "second opinion" be obtained for (1) any surgical procedure destroying brain tissue or (2) the surgical implantation of hormones to reduce male sexual drive; and consent *or* a second opinion for (1) electroconvulsive therapy or (2) medication (during detention of a patient for treatment of a mental disorder) for over three months.

Two recent cases in English courts, *Sidaway v. Bethlem Royal Hospital Governors and others*, and *Freeman v. Home Office*, deal specifically with the issue of informed consent in English law. Mrs. Sidaway had an operation on her spinal cord in 1974 to relieve pain in her neck, shoulder, and arm. During the operation the arteries of the spinal cord were damaged and this resulted in damage to the cord itself, leading to severe impairment of movement in her right arm and leg. She brought an action for negligence on the grounds that the surgeon had been in breach of his duty because he had failed to warn her of all the possible risks inherent in the operation so that she had not been in a position to give informed consent to the operation.[20]

Mr. Freeman was serving life imprisonment, during which time he was prescribed major tranquilizers both orally and by injection. He brought an action for trespass of the person on the grounds that the drugs were administered without his consent. He argued that for a patient's consent to be operative in law it had to be 'informed' and that the patient had to be informed of (1) what he was suffering from, (2) the precise nature of the treatment being proposed, and (3) what, if any, adverse effects and risks were involved in the treatment.

Both cases were heard in appeal and dismissed, *Sidaway* being the precedent for *Freeman*. The issue dealt with in the *Sidaway* case was how much information a doctor is required to give a patient. Mrs. Sidaway was told of the possibility of damage to the nerve roots, but not of the more remote possibility of damage to the blood vessels and cord itself. It was determined that a doctor was under a general duty to disclose such information as was reasonable to enable the patient to make a rational choice whether to agree to or refuse a proposed treatment, but that the doctrine of informed consent, based on full disclosure of all the facts to the patient, was not the appropriate test in English law.

This position was stated rather forcefully and in a way that might be misunderstood, in Dunn's opinion: "The doctrine of 'informed consent' forms no part of English law."[21] His reasons, however, are quite clear and go to the heart of the controversy:

> The evidence in this case showed that a contrary result would be damaging to the relationship of trust and confidence between doctor and patient, and might well have an adverse effect on the practice of medicine. It is doubtful whether it

would be of any significant benefit to patients, most of whom prefer to put themselves unreservedly in the hands of their doctors. This is not in my view "paternalism," to repeat an evocative word used in argument. It is simply an acceptance of the doctor/patient relationship as it has developed in this country. The principal effect of accepting the proposition advanced by the plaintiff would be likely to be an increase in the number of claims for professional negligence against doctors. This would be likely to have an adverse effect on the general standards of medical care, since doctors would inevitably be concerned to safeguard themselves against such claims, rather than to concentrate on their primary duty of treating their patients.[22]

The *Freeman* case involves the issue of psychiatric treatment, but the case is more interesting for the questions it raises than for the issues it settles since it was determined that consent must in fact have occurred:

Since the doctrine of informed consent formed no part of English law, the sole issue was whether on the facts the plaintiff had consented to the administration of the drugs and on that issue the trial judge had found that the plaintiff had so consented.[23]

The issues of the right of a nonautonomous prisoner or involuntary psychiatric patient to refuse a treatment are complex. Reference is made in the *Freeman* decision both to the Nuremberg standards and to the relevant section of the Mental Health Act 1983, as well as including a telling reference to American law. Sir John Donaldson notes in his opinion that "the American doctrine of 'informed consent' has no place in the law of England."[24] While informed consent is not a uniquely American concept, the comparison is worth making. Informed consent is an attempt to focus particular attention on the rights of individuals, which is an essential cornerstone of democracy. However, if the limits of those rights are also not appreciated it is possible for an individual in effect to hold the state or the society hostage in exercising those rights. At some point the rights of individuals infringe on the freedoms of others, and a line must be drawn as is sometimes the case with prisoners and involuntarily detained psychiatric patients. The negligence awards Dunn worried about might be another such example. In the United States, it is routine for neurosurgeons in some states to carry annual malpractice insurance premiums in excess of Mrs. Sidaway's calculated damages (£67,000). This malpractice crisis is a crisis of confidence that England and other countries would do well to avoid.

Yet there is a difference between the absolute requirement to determine after the fact what a particular doctor should have disclosed and the choices a particular physician might make in striving to promote trust with a particular patient. The dilemma between autonomy and the need for some degree of paternalism is inescapable. The regulatory guidelines set forth in statutes such as the Mental Health Act 1983 or in precedents such as the *Sidaway* and *Freeman* decisions are necessary but not sufficient for the highest ethical standards toward which a physician should aspire. It is therefore important not only to keep the provisions of the law in mind, but also to remember the ethical principles that underlie the legal requirements.

INFORMED CONSENT IN SWEDEN

Sweden has enacted some of the most socially progressive legislation in the world with regard to the rights and welfare of its citizens. It is therefore particularly informative to consider a conflict that emerged in Gothenburg concerning objections to the paternalistic attitudes of surgeons there who refused to make available to women the breast-sparing "lumpectomy" in place of the traditional mastectomy. In a confrontation that received substantial attention by the news media, a sizable group of women in Gothenburg insisted that the choice of operation should be the patient's instead of the doctor's.

The surgeons argued that the efficacy of the breast-sparing operation, the so-called Ludwig procedure, had not been established and therefore the doctor was required to make the decision as to the best treatment available. Upon persistent pressure, a randomized controlled trial was undertaken, assigning patients to three groups, mastectomy, Ludwig procedure, or no treatment. Consent was not solicited for this randomization because under a little-known clause of the Helsinki modification of the Geneva accords, consent may be dispensed with if it is felt that requiring consent would cause undue anxiety.

It should be quickly pointed out that Department of Health and Human Services guidelines regulating informed consent would not permit this loophole to be employed in the United States. It should also be noted that the concept of informed consent as we have come to understand it, respecting the autonomy and even the rights of patients, does not give patients the right to require treatments that the doctor does not judge to be effective. What makes the Gothenburg situation informative is the idea that the locus of decision making should reside either with the doctor or the patient, not in a partnership ongoing in time. We could conceive of a complete transformation of medicine into a commodity in which any provider might provide a service for which there was a demand in the market. This would be a radical departure from the idea of professional stewardship.

One other feature of the Swedish system is worthy of reflection. In a socialized medical system, the doctor is not in fact working for the patient directly but for the state. The doctor is charged with the welfare of the population, not necessarily with the interests of the individual. The confrontation as it emerged was a confrontation of groups rather than individuals, played out in a public arena, rather than in private, confidential relationships where there might have been the prospect of resolution.

INFORMED CONSENT IN JAPAN AND THE ASIAN PACIFIC

The Declaration of Geneva is a remarkable document in that it was signed by most nations of the world—Western, Eastern, First World, Communist, Third World. The broad principles of human rights are ones that most peoples could and have agreed to, in stark contrast to the universally condemned atrocities of the Nazi government. This broad consensus obscures some of the more subtle contours of cultural difference that we are now beginning to appreciate.

We now hear from colleagues in Asian Pacific countries that although the Declaration of Geneva was signed, its emphasis on individuality does not reflect the values of some cultural groups, which emphasize more the community solidarity and the authority of chiefs or elders to decide for family or tribe.

In the Philippines, for example, family ties and the traditional Philippines system of reciprocal obligations between individuals, known as *utang na loob* (literally, inner debt), exist in a constant loose tension with the strivings for a Western-style modern democracy. While those schooled in the liberties of Western-style democracy might judge such a network of obligations as "backward," we also should be mindful of the disintegration of social fabric that can occur in a society with unlimited pursuit of individual self-interest, pleasure, and liberty.

In Japan, which in many ways is adopting increasingly a Westernized emphasis on individual rights, old notions of deference to paternalistic authority still exist. For many years in Japan, the patient or his family have been requested to sign a type of consent form before surgical operations are performed in hospitals. However, the traditional Japanese consent form was not based on the rights of the individual, but rather served as a waiver in advance by patients of their right to sue for damages, even if the doctor was negligent. It read, "I, a patient, and my family promise that we will never complain of any injury incurred during treatment."[25]

Two suits in the 1970s have begun to establish the principle of rights of the individual patient. Both involved claims against surgeons for operations without consent, and in both cases the patients recovered monetary awards. In one suit an actress consented to removal of the right breast because of cancer in the mammary glands. During the operation the surgeon examined the left breast and determined that a mass there might subsequently become cancerous and that it too should be removed. He did so without specifically obtaining consent.

The second case involved an operation for a cancer of the tongue. The patient was not told the diagnosis, but simply was told that resection of the tongue was recommended. The patient did not agree to it, and the doctor barely managed to convince the patient by explaining that the disease was an ulcer and the ulcerated part was to be cauterized. The doctor then proceeded to resect approximately one-third of the tongue.

These two cases have brought about an increased emphasis on obtaining written consent in Japan, though many of the consent forms still contain the exemption clause, "I, the patient, will make no complaint at all against the result of the medical treatment," even though legal authorities in Japan have commented that such a clause is meaningless and void.[26]

INFORMED CONSENT BEHIND THE IRON CURTAIN

Even in the West certain liberties are curtailed. The manic may be constrained from wildly spending his money, the depressed person from harming himself, the schizophrenic from harming someone else. Under the watchful eye of civil libertarians, we recognize the need to restrict certain freedoms. Yet even the most paternalistic of physicians recognizes that freedom of political expression should not be curtailed. The practice in Eastern-bloc countries of psychiatrically detaining political dissidents has received widespread and vigorous opposition in the West. Two points need to be appreciated from the standpoint of our consideration of informed consent.

First, the opposition to physicians' cooperation with the government in the detention of political dissidents is a political issue reflecting culturally based values that are believed in with fervor and universal intent. They are rooted in deeply held convictions, and their goal is not merely the alteration of medical practices but the alteration of a political system that does not respect the same principles and concept of human dignity.

Second, the condemnation of that cooperation is based on grounds that are claimed to be universal to the medical profession, independent of the political system in which the physician may be operating. It is an attempt to place ethics, in this case professional ethics, on a plane different from and above the law, which may be subject to political expediency. Those who would argue for the abandonment of the Hippocratic tradition of the physician being held to a higher standard of conduct by virtue of professional commitment should be careful not to take individual freedom too much for granted. It is something that must be guarded with vigilance.

INFORMED CONSENT AND TORTURE

A related but slightly different issue is that of physicians who cooperate with military governments in torture. Physicians not only administer torture on occasion but more commonly examine patients to see if they can tolerate more torture. Such blatant abuses of not only informed consent but much more basic concepts of human rights and dignity are, to say the least, horrific to contemplate. The coercion of not only the political prisoners but also the physicians must pose excruciating agony for all but the most cynical and misguided physicians involved. There is no need even to debate whether such activities are unethical. Our consideration here is to consider their implications for professional definition.

An example sets the consideration: The ethics committee of the São Paulo Medical Society meets weekly to review hundreds of allegations of unethical conduct by physicians, some of which involved cooperation with the military government in torturing prisoners. In Brazil the ethics committee has statutory authority as an arm of the government to impose its sanctions, unlike the voluntary professional societies, which are sometimes criticized for not having sufficient power to discipline their members. To the ethics committee in São Paulo there was no question that cooperation with torture was unethical, and it duly imposed appropriate sanctions against physicians who were found to be involved. However, since the government (in this case the recent military government) had authority over the regulation of physicians, it was able to prevent the sanctions from being imposed.

This sobering example deserves consideration because it helps to dramatize a situation far removed from the kinds of considerations we usually apply to issues of professional regulation. It speaks in its extremity to the importance of the sphere of professional autonomy as providing an ethical perspective on professional regulation different from the interests that a state might impose, subject to the limitations of the political process. Just as there are very good reasons for maintaining the separation of church and state, so also there are good reasons for maintaining the separation of the ethical aspects of profession from the current whims of the political process.

CONCLUSION

Informed consent serves to focus our thinking and practice on the ethical dimensions of our medical and scientific procedures involving human beings. The focus on informed consent forces us to rethink our value of rationality, our tradition of intellectual clarity, the ambiguities of language, and how we deal with ambivalent affects. In so doing, we could decide to isolate those dissimilar from ourselves by an arbitrary division into autonomous and nonautonomous persons. Or we might come to recognize something of ourselves in the psychiatric patients with whom we are concerned. This may be a humbling experience, especially if our concept of ourselves has tended to stress the cognitive side of our being, but it may be a humanizing experience as well. The view of informed consent stressed here emphasizes the relatedness of people more than their autonomy. This approach brings us into closer proximity with human suffering than may be comfortable, but it seems at least a minimum ethical requirement for participation in those procedures for which we have come to expect an informed consent.

The ethical norms of a psychiatrist employing a psychodynamic approach serve as a reminder that principles other than autonomy are worthy of consideration. To achieve the proper balance between best interest and autonomy, one must know the patient, a task that requires time and an ongoing relationship. The more encompassing principle of partnership may ameliorate the shortcomings of the principles of both beneficence and autonomy. The approach of the psychiatrist, far from being inadequate, suggests a useful model for all physicians and investigators: Take the time to know the patient (or experimental subject) as a person.

CHAPTER 7

THE PLACE OF VIRTUE AND CHARACTER IN ETHICS: PSYCHIATRY'S CONTRIBUTION TO ETHICS

THE REDISCOVERY of virtue and character as concepts worthy of consideration in medical ethics is welcome indeed. The field of medical ethics and what has come to be known as bioethics have been severely handicapped without these concepts. The concept of virtue restores a lost dimension to medical ethics. In the past decade or two, medical ethics has become a very impersonal enterprise, all but ignoring the moral psychology of moral agents (both physicians and patients) who must make decisions. An analysis of virtues in the immediacy of the clinical setting offers a texture to moral life that an analysis of neither moral rules nor utilities can offer.

In the following passages, I suggest that the concepts of virtue and character are fundamental to understanding what a profession such as medicine really is. Furthermore, the prevailing view of professions, which defines professions primarily in terms of technical skills and promotion of self-interest, fails to appreciate this. The prevailing accounts of ethics, lacking an adequately developed moral psychology and ignoring considerations of virtue and character, have failed to set the matter straight.

Roger Sider and Colleen Clements, a psychiatrist-philosopher team, have elaborated these problems in an important article, "Psychiatry's Contribution to Medical Ethics Education,"[1] the title of which I have adapted for use in this chapter. They note that medical ethics has not generally involved an interaction between medicine and ethics, but a superimposition of traditional philosophical categories on the clinical setting. To redress this imbalance, they suggest employing needed aspects of psychiatric thought to shape ethical thought and action in medical ethics education. They suggest three components of ethics education of which psychiatrists have special knowledge: (1) affective components of rationality, (2) the developmental perspective, and (3) the professional ethos. Sider and Clements note the following:

99

Psychodynamic awareness has helped us to see that motives to observe as well as to violate moral precepts are often deeply conflicted and highly irrational, yet powerfully persuasive. Particularly in the concrete setting of the office or clinic, ethical reasoning may rapidly give way to unethical rationalization. It is surprising that so little attention is paid to this problem in the current literature on ethics education, as if man, the reasoning animal, were not simultaneously possessed of powerful passions and appetites. Ethics education must include, then, the juxtaposition of the results of rational ethical reflection with equally important nonrational factors in the physician such as sensitivity, compassion, capacity for social bonding, and quality of object relations. It is only here, as reason conjoins affect and attitude, that the learning of ethics as an aspect of clinical practice can begin. This complex educational process is largely one of learning about oneself or, more precisely, what is revealed and evoked in oneself as a function of the clinical role [or responsibilities].

In other words, psychiatry picks up where modern philosophy abandoned the ancient admonition to "Know thyself." Modern philosophy, having appreciated the sterility of the Cartesian-Baconian epistemological scheme as played out in logical positivism, is beginning to look again to the considerations of virtue and character. This chapter and the following one develop these considerations in greater detail in light of problems faced by the practicing physician and those people who turn to members of the medical profession for help.

MORAL AND THERAPEUTIC CONSIDERATIONS OF CHARACATER

The concept of character occupies a central position in psychoanalysis and psychodynamic psychotherapy. Character also occupies a central position in the lexicon of moral philosophy. It is usually held that the technical use of the term "character" has little relationship to the ordinary use, which has moral connotations. Psychotherapies are overtly value-neutral or at least nonjudgmental, whereas moral philosophy is avowedly judgmental or at least reflective on value judgments. There is, nonetheless, an important conjunction between these various uses of the term "character." The psychoanalytic consideration of character, which is concerned with the development of morality, is just as relevant to moral philosophy and everyday morality as it is to medical considerations in the treatment of "character disorders" or "personality disorders."

Freud's earliest reference to "character" belies the judgmental connotation that is associated with the term. In 1904 Freud observed: "If the physician has to deal with a worthless character, he soon loses the interest which makes it possible for him to enter profoundly into the patient's mental life. Deep rooted malformations of character, traits of an actually degenerate constitution, show themselves during treatment as sources of a resistance that can scarcely be overcome."[2]

Moral philosophers are showing renewed interest in the concept of character, which stems in part from a recognition that moral propositions do not address the problems that motivate ethical reflection. It is not enough to consider what people say about what is right, it is also necessary to be concerned with what people actually do. Thus many philosophers have developed a renewed interest in the Aristotelian concern with "the virtues." Erich Fromm notes that it is "the virtuous or vicious character, rather than the (particular) virtues or vices, which is the true subject matter of ethical inquiry."[3]

Implicit and explicit ideas of character provide the rationale for attempts at shaping and molding the behavior of successive generations. Parents set limits, instill ideals, and consciously and unconsciously manipulate shame and guilt according to notions of what is right and good. Schools extend this parental function, and to the extent that widespread agreement exists on certain values, it is possible to discern patterns of culture, sometimes referred to as "national character." The English public schools, for example, developed in the nineteenth century renewed interest in the ideals of chivalry as the proper form of education for the English gentleman. Virtues of order, self-restraint, mutual dependence, and heroic and generous actions were instilled as much through games (sports) as exhortations. Historian Girouard has noted that "Character more than scholarship was the aim of [the] teaching."[4] The *Encyclopaedia Britannica* says of the Rugby School under Thomas Arnold that "it became not merely a place where a certain amount of classical or general learning was to be obtained, but a sphere of intellectual, moral and religious discipline, where healthy characters were formed, and men were trained for the duties, struggles and responsibilities of life."[5]

CHARACTER AS CHARACTERISTIC

Often the term "character" is used to speak of those traits that are characteristic of a particular individual. One might say, "That's just like Mary," or "You could expect that of her," or "John walks just like his father," or "He has the same patterns of speech." This use of character refers to a certain predictability. It is morally neutral, though of course value judgments may be made about another's characteristics, especially certain traits such as honesty or courage. Character in this sense may involve certain unconscious identifications made in childhood and may be closely related to the complex processes involved in formation of "identity" or "personality."

This view of character may seem at first glance to be at variance with the moral connotation, but careful consideration should demonstrate that there is more convergence than might be apparent. Those traits that are most characteristic and consistent are what distinguish that particular individual; that is, form his identity and make him unique. It is on the basis of such character traits that one is known and judged by others. If the judgment is favorable, one is spoken of as having character or a good character or as having integrity.

CHARACTER AS RESISTANCE

The psychoanalytic use of the term "character" designates the more or less fixed and permanent resistances to recovering unconscious memories of childhood experiences. Character in this sense is what prevents the uncovering of the unconscious or gets in the way of treatment.

An important early distinction in the psychoanalytic literature was made between symptom neuroses and character neuroses. Early psychoanalytic treatment focused on the treatment of those symptoms, notably hysterical conversion symptoms, phobias, and compulsions (with anxiety and depression added to the list of symptoms). Gradually this pattern has shifted to the present situation, in which those presenting for psychoanalytic treatment are more likely to have character neuroses. Symptom neuroses are ego-dystonic; they make the person uncomfortable. Character neuroses are by definition ego-syntonic: The character is the self, the person, the ego, the identity. The character neurotic may make others uncomfortable and thus have difficulty in forming and sustaining intimate relationships. Whereas conflict is the essence of neurosis, there is a relative absence of conflict in the formation of character.

DEVELOPMENT OF THE PSYCHOANALYTIC THEORY OF CHARACTER

Freud initially considered character as an impulse, akin to the libido. In the *Interpretation of Dreams* (1900) he notes: "What we describe as our 'character' is based on the memory traces of our impressions; and, moreover, the impressions which have had the greatest effect on us—those of our earliest growth—are precisely the ones which scarcely ever become conscious."[6]

In stressing the importance of childhood sexuality, Freud stressed the essential normality of the child in dealing with sexual feelings and fantasies. In "Three Essays on the Theory of Sexuality," he notes that "the multifariously perverse sexual disposition of childhood can accordingly be regarded as the source of a number of our virtues insofar as through reaction-formation it stimulates their development."[7]

If the idea that the virtues are stimulated by perverse childhood impulses seems paradoxical, it is probably less so than Freud's 1908 paper on "Character and Anal Erotism," where he notes that in people with prominent character traits of orderliness, parsimony, and obstinacy, there regularly turns out to be also a preponderance of concerns with the anal region and with the feeling and circumstances surrounding defecation.[8] Those likely to consider themselves most virtuous are those who are best defended against the affects associated with the anal period.

Abraham built on these ideas in his "Contributions to the Theory of the Anal Character."[9] He distinguished the retentive and eliminative modes. He noted traits of cleanliness and orderliness, of pleasure in production and in achievement, a tendency toward obedience and yielding to others, an exaggerated sense of autonomy, difficulty in giving things away, making presents, paying money, a desire to control others and to make them dependent, a tendency toward negativism and opposition. He began to elaborate phenomenological descriptions of particular character traits. The obsessional neurotics in particular manifested these "anal" traits, but tended to be relatively free of conflict about them. (See also Freud, 1913.[10])

An important contribution of Freud in 1915 was the introduction of the notion of character as resistance, a notion that Reich elaborated in his discussion of "character armour."[11] Reich assumed that at any time when, due to external factors such as the repressive intervention of parental figures, anxiety over sexual drives is aroused, the child masters his "infantile phobia" by turning some of these very drives to defensive purposes. At the same time there occurs an identification with the repressive and inhibiting aspect of the parental figure.

In the treatment of neurotics, the analyst is interested in the drives, but the analyst meets resistance to uncovering drives posed by the patient's character. Thus character is a defense in that it protects the individual against unpleasant affects. Or it is a resistance encountered when the analyst and patient seek to uncover what is being defended against.

CHARACTER AND MORAL DEVELOPMENT

What about the moral sense of character? Is character armour what the philosopher has in mind in speaking of character? Appreciating character in developmental terms makes one perhaps more tolerant and less judgmental about it. It becomes easier to appreciate why people are the way they are when we understand what they have experienced and how it may be similar to what all people have to cope with in their own emotional development. Certainly it is easier to empathize with the patient.

But tolerance is not the main consideration either, and psychoanalysis in its developmental framework provides a basis for judging character. One may tolerate and empathize with developmental aberration in treatment, but there is the implicit expectation that the patient will adhere to the therapeutic goal of greater maturity through rational understanding.

Maturity is the hallmark of character in developmental consideration. This means that the person largely has resolved conflicts over dependency, control, dominance, and submission and seeing others narcissistically only in terms of gratifications provided or not provided; has reached the genital level of development; and has resolved the Oedipus complex. Once one has

103

realized and accepted that the parent of the opposite sex is unattainable and that one must make one's own way in the world outside the family, one is free, as Freud put it, to love and work. It is at this stage that the efforts of the moral philosopher can become effective. When a person can accept his place in a world of which he is not the center, he can appreciate the quest for principles that go beyond himself, a categorical imperative, a Golden Rule. It requires a certain maturity, which age itself may not provide, to act on principles that are not rigidly determined or compulsively driven.

THE PSYCHOANALYTIC TREATMENT OF CHARACTER DISORDERS

Value judgments are inescapable when considering the treatment of character disturbances, such as the paranoid, schizoid, histrionic, narcissistic, antisocial, borderline, avoidant, dependent, compulsive, and passive-aggressive (to use the *Diagnostic and Statistical Manual of Mental Disorders, Third Edition [DSM-III]* categorization of personality disorders) or "Those Wrecked by Success," "Criminals Out of a Sense of Guilt," "The Exceptions," and the "Aristocratic Character," to identify some of the character-types described in the literature. [12]

In calling these character-types "personality disorders," a judgment is made, presumably by the diagnosing psychiatrist but possibly by a family member or someone who finds the behavior disturbing, that a disorder is present. *DSM-III*, in its attempt to remain uncommited to any single theory of character, incorrectly indicates that no information is available about the etiology of these disorders, which is not strictly true unless one is willing to ignore developmental evidence. In the United Kingdom the definition of "mental disorder" under the Mental Health Act 1983 includes "arrested or incomplete development of mind" as well as "mental illness and psychopathic disorder." *DSM-III* avoids developmental considerations in order to remain descriptive and unbiased toward any particular theory of character.

Insofar as the character pathology represents a defense against an underlying anxiety (that is, an underlying neurosis), then it is likely to be amenable to psychoanalytic treatment. The principle is to convert the character pathology into a neurosis by confronting it, making the ego-syntonic aspects ego-dystonic or ego-alien. One must analyze the character traits before the infantile sexual conflict; one must analyze resistance before content. [13] Auchincloss and Michels have commented on this process:

> Psychoanalytic clinicians have always taken a seemingly contrary stance toward their patients' descriptions of their problems. If the patient describes ego-alien symptoms, the therapist attempts to demonstrate that the symptoms are not really alien but reflect unconscious themes central to his mental life. On the other hand, if the patient presents ego-syntonic character pathology, the analyst spends a great deal of time trying to weaken the patient's unquestioning

acceptance of these character patterns by driving a wedge between the character pathology and that part of the patient that is capable of self-observation. The attempt is to make character ego-alien, at least to the extent that the patient can observe it and analyze it, whether or not he ultimately reclaims it as his own.[14]

There is potential danger in ignoring the character defenses. That danger is treating the character-disordered person as a neurotic. Treatment may go much more smoothly initially if the therapist does not confront character defenses and accepts what the patient says about how badly the world has treated him. Marital troubles are because of the spouse, and the parents are always to blame. The therapist thus places himself in the role of the helpful, good parent, to whom the patient can express positive feelings but never negative ones.

Conversely, challenging the presented view of reality, however gently, may cause anger and resentment. But it also offers the potential for growth and development when transference distortions are clarified. It is such crucial moments in therapy that offer opportunities for insight and understanding. Though they may seem to depart from a supportive stance, the support of the therapeutic relationship is really what makes it possible to look at painful life experiences.

François Truffaut brilliantly illustrates what disastrous consequences can occur when one fails to assess character and character defenses in his film *Une Belle Femme Comme Moi* (English title: *Such a Gorgeous Kid*). Here the naive hero who identifies with his subject is a sociologist studying a sociopathic woman, whose problems he discovers come from her unfortunate childhood. She has killed her father, but he deserved it, she tells our hero: He tried to rape her when she was 15. Taken in by her story, the sociologist makes excuses for her, first to the authorities and then to the news media. He never questions his own relationship with her until finally he has won her release from prison, but by then he has become an accomplice to her schemes and ends up behind bars himself.

The confrontation of character pathology immediately raises ethical questions for the analyst. Does the person really want to change and how much? Is this not an assault on the person's autonomy and freedom of choice? These are not frivolous questions because it is possible to be heavy-handed in the delicate transference relationship and to influence the patient unduly with one's own values. This is why the countertransference must constantly be scrutinized. But they are not questions that can be dismissed by putting all the responsibility on the patient to say what he wants. That is because the patient's unconscious wishes and desires need to be considered, and in order to be considered, they need to be brought to consciousness. This is what is really meant by autonomy, and it is in this sense that increased autonomy is the goal of analysis.

The philosopher Abraham Kaplan has assessed the moral situation of psychoanalysis very nicely: "Psychoanalysis allots less freedom than man thought he had, but makes possible more freedom than in fact he had."[15]

Viewed in the developmental perspective, the personality disorders receive a negative character judgment, not because helping professionals place themselves in the position of judging other people's characters, except insofar as people ask for help, but because such disorders represent a loss of potentiality, a destruction of the self, and often an imposition on others.

The psychoanalytic concept of character thus applies to a particular technical issue in the conduct of psychoanalytic treatment, which would seem at first to be unrelated to the moral connotations of character. However, if one considers the moral implications of development toward maturity, the psychoanalytic concept of character comes much closer to the usual considerations of morality and further suggests a basis by which character may be judged.

It is worth noting that not all judgments of character are necessarily moral. Calling something right does not necessarily make it so. Polanyi has called our attention to the way in which judgments of morality may actually reflect a "moral inversion" in which the claim to morality is used as a way of capturing power and influence.[16] One example of a claim to morality that clearly does not constitute moral maturity is the moralistic outlook of the obsessional character. The traits of orderliness, rationality, and punctuality —often piously held—may be defenses against the underlying shame of the anal period. The so-called authoritarian personality falls into this category and has accepted the punitive strictures of parents in a morally sadistic way, intent on controlling others but lacking the flexibility to weigh, assess, and make value judgments in a particular context.

To bring the wheel full circle, we should note that much of what passes for ethical reflection may fall into this category, attempting to deduce abstract moral rules that foreclose on the necessity of moral agents actually having to make decisions in morally ambiguous situations. The psychoanalyst and the moral philosopher would probably agree that the person of character would be the mature person who could make responsible decisions in complex situations.

THE IMPORTANCE OF VIRTUE IN PROFESSIONAL GATEKEEPING

A profession, defined by its ethics and the shared commitment of its members to an ideal of service, must attend carefully to what sort of person is allowed to assume the responsibilities and accompanying privileges of professional activity. The determination of who shall be accepted into the profession and the monitoring of the performance of the members of the profession is an important responsibility of professional organizations. The control of entry and exit has been traditionally considered to be an important function for professional self-regulation. Leaving aside for a moment the question of who holds the responsibility for such regulation, I wish to establish that such activities are essential to the idea of a profession and that they are impossible to fulfill without some concept of virtue. If medicine is more than just technical expertise, then some understanding of virtue or "character" is essential to what we expect of a physician whether we acknowledge it explicitly or not. It is not sufficient that a physician, for example, be knowledgeable about matters of physiology and biochemistry: That physician must also be able to communicate with patients and adhere to certain standards of ethics.

Entry decisions are made quite formally in the United States with medical school admissions (since we graduate almost all the students we admit). Most admissions committees look for students who are not only academically competent but who also possess some measure of the requisite virtues. Though the vocabulary for talking about requisite virtues has largely atrophied and the emphasis is placed on grades and board scores, which can be readily quantified, I believe most admissions committees retain some sense of trying to select candidates for medical education who will make "good doctors." I suggest that some concept of virtue is at work even though it usually functions at a tacit level of awareness. Efforts to bring these considerations into explicit focus should only enhance their legitimacy and prominence.

The control of exit from professions is a responsibility variously held by state licensing bodies and professional organizations. The state licensing boards, which have the power to grant licenses, also have the power to rescind them. Professional organizations such as the AMA and various specialty organizations can and do expel members from their organizations if they fail to live up to the standards of ethics. There is a widely held perception that professional organizations are reluctant to move against their members, but in the past 15 years professional organizations have become increasingly aware of the necessity to "police their own." The AMA's Council on Mental Health, for example, introduced a model impaired-physician statute that has subsequently been adopted by most states, which makes provisions for the licensing boards to review the license of any physician thought to be disabled by virtue of physical or mental illness or substance abuse and to provide legal protection for the whistle-blower. Again a concept of virtue is in operation in such considerations, for the model statute provides for a humane "therapeutic" intervention while maintaining the necessity of professional "discipline."

Another example of this kind of activity is the increased emphasis of professional organizations on investigating grievances of dissatisfied patients. The activities of the American Psychiatric Association's (APA's) Ethics Committee is an example of this kind of activity. In 1973 APA adopted "Annotations Especially Applicable to Psychiatry" as an addition to the AMA's *Principles of Medical Ethics*.[17] Each member of the APA is expected to be familiar with this statement of ethical principles, and it serves as a reference for any complaint of unethical conduct brought against a member.

While sociologists and antitrust theorists might argue that such activities primarily serve the economic interests of the members of the professional group, such gatekeeping activities serve the public interest as well by assuring that certain standards of professional competence and integrity are maintained.

THE CENTRAL VIRTUES OF THE MEDICAL PROFESSION

Thus far I have argued that a concept of virtue is central to the idea of a profession; that moral discourse has been largely handicapped without explicit acknowledgment of the concept of virtue; that the concept is implicit in the activities of professional organizations; and that a potentially destructive aspect of the field of medical ethics (bioethics) is that it has been operating in a cultural and psychological void as if there were no such thing as virtue or a moral agent. One might reasonably expect now a catalog of appropriate medical virtues, virtues appropriate to our contemporary culture or to the culture of medicine. I am prepared to offer at least a start on such a catalogue by suggesting two virtues that have been central to the traditional ideals of a profession: trustworthiness and respect for confidentiality.

The notion of trustworthiness is a constant theme throughout the various articulated codes of ethics from the Hippocratic Oath through Percival's *Medical Ethics* to the various revisions of the AMA codes. The physician should be someone whom the patient can trust and someone who inspires the confidence of the patient. Perhaps in ancient times even more so than in modern times, this was important because the inspiration of trust in the physician, confidence in the treatment, and hope for improvement were essential to the success of the treatment when the physician had little to offer. In the contemporary era, physiological interventions can be much more specific, but the personal ministrations of the physician to the patient remain, I believe, an indispensable part of medical practice. Knowledge is always incomplete and technical power limited.

There is perhaps an even more basic reason for suggesting that trustworthiness is an essential virtue for the medical profession. That is the psychological primacy of trust as a basic human quality, really the first issue in psychological development with which the newborn and its caretakers must deal. It has been demonstrated that consistency in the nurturing environment, that is, predictability that the parents will meet the infant's needs, has been shown to leave one with a sense of trust in the world and the ability to trust others; absence of such consistency in early childhood leaves one always potentially uncertain and in doubt. It may seem a large jump to draw an analogy between the child and the patient (perhaps an adult, autonomous, and rational creature), but there is a fundamental way in which one is quite dependent on the physician when one seeks help. The overlays of adult rationality in no way significantly lessen the psychological significance of that supplication in time of need. The patient needs to know that the physician will not do anything to violate that sense of confidence and expectation that help will indeed be rendered.

The second virtue I believe is related to the first: respect for confidentiality. Again the tradition of confidentiality has an ancient heritage, going back at least to medieval common law traditions, which protected the confidentiality of communications with a physician, lawyer, or clergyman. The psychological reasons for this are evident. One cannot freely disclose to the physician or other professional the relevant information (history) that will be needed to make an assessment of the problem and render help unless one knows that that communication is private and not to be disclosed elsewhere. This virtue of respect for confidentiality is particularly relevant in the modern era because so much of medical care is delivered by teams, often including nonprofessionals, and because of the difficulty of protecting the contents of medical records.

THE VIRTUES OF THE PATIENT

It might seem a bit out of place to consider the virtues of the patient when the popular sentiment seems so much to view the patient as passive in front of the overwhelming power of the professional. Nineteenth-century statements such as Percival's code and the early versions of the AMA codes spoke of the responsibilities of the patient to the physician, especially duties such as loyalty, which clearly seem antiquated. If any sense of mutuality of the doctor-patient relationship is to be maintained (or restored), it is reasonable to think of the virtues of the patient.

Again trustworthiness might head the list. Honesty might be a central consideration of such trustworthiness, especially in terms of forthrightness in the disclosure of information that might be relevant to the physician's understanding of the problems for which the patient is seeking help. This is particularly important in sorting out those problems that have a psychosomatic component—and this probably includes a much greater proportion of patient-physician encounters than we generally acknowledge. Furthermore, we are increasingly coming to consider the responsibilities of patients in health matters that involve lifestyle, especially health problems arising from alcohol and tobacco, improper diet, or bad habits (such as insufficient exercise). The physician can treat alcoholic gastritis, for example, but the patient and ultimately the community must accept some responsibility for the treatment of the alcoholic and alcoholism. Still a social judgment is involved in shifting concepts of disease and illness, which are increasingly medicalized or demedicalized: abortion, child abuse, homosexuality as perversion or alternate sexual preference, hypertension, hysterical conversion, malingering, passive-dependency, and other so-called personality disorders. A sophisticated appreciation of all these potentially medical problems is really impossible without recourse to some concept of virtue.

CONCLUSION

Two divergent approaches to ethics—bioethics and professional ethics—have appeared in recent years to be at cross-purposes. What I am suggesting here is that both have been handicapped without recourse to the concept of virtue. Ultimately what is at stake is a rethinking of cultural values, notions of the responsibility of individuals in a society to one another, the relationships of members of a family and community, and the relationships of professionals with those served. While a chapter of this scope cannot attempt to solve these various cultural issues, I think it can be demonstrated that the concept of virtue in ethics is a legitimate starting point for resolving some of the misunderstandings that have characterized ethics for the past several years.

CHAPTER 8

IDEALISM IN MEDICAL ETHICS: THE PURSUIT OF MORAL PERFECTION

THE SELF AS MORAL AGENT

There is an equivocation in modern philosophy that makes ethics a problematic undertaking. It stems from our ability to give impersonal accounts of human behavior, the things people do, while at the same time experiencing ourselves as participants in history. So accustomed have we become to looking at ourselves from an imaginary point outside ourselves and outside our world that we often forget who we are; we forget that thread of history that makes us uniquely ourselves. We could never tolerate a complete dissociation from the circumstances of our existence and maintain our sanity, yet a selective surrender to the forces of impersonality can from time to time be a convenient escape from the awesome responsibilities that are a part of the human condition.

A theory of ethics must speak to this equivocation. One may look at ethics from the perspective of the self, the person, the agent who must decide and act in a social context (upwards perspective), or one may look at ethics from the perspective of the social order into which the individual must fit (downwards perspective). The questions that one formulates for ethics may be very different in these two perspectives. It is even possible to divert one's attention away from the self by abstractly formulating the questions for the ethical undertaking, yet the self never disappears no matter how impersonal the considerations become. "What is right or wrong?" is a very different question from "What ought I do?" Yet both are properly considered ethical questions. What is not proper is to consider one approach exclusive of the other. The distinction between absolutist and relativistic ethics is itself specious, suggesting that it may be possible and appropriate to ignore either the person or the context. This tension, which has plagued modern philosophy since the Enlightenment, leaves us believing that we must make a choice—adherence to ourselves or to an objective reality—when in fact we need to understand how to locate ourselves in a reality that is beyond ourselves.

The recognition of multiple tasks for ethical reflection, which are inclusive and not exclusive, raises questions about the methods of thought that may be appropriate and helpful in studying ethics. When is a question or issue understood to be an ethical question or issue? Does saying that it must be personal mean that it depends on one's perspective? If so, is this to suggest that different conclusions could be reached in different situations? If not, could one hope for an absolute guideline as a point of reference in making decisions?

> But after all, what is goodness? Answer me that, Alexey. Goodness is one thing with me and another with a Chinaman, so it's a relative thing. Or isn't it? Is it not relative? A treacherous question! You won't laugh if I tell you it's kept me awake two nights. I only wonder now how people can live and think nothing of it. Vanity![1]

The abstractly formulated question "What is goodness?" is not the way ethical dilemmas are usually experienced. They emerge from the context of the lives we lead. It is in an attempt to get away from the immediacy of the decisions we must make that we abstractly formulate our question, so that we may act with less turmoil than Ivan Karamazov experienced. People can live and think nothing of the question because action is often taken without the intense reflection that perplexes Dostoevsky's characters. At the one extreme are those impulsive characters who reflect not at all on their actions; at the other extreme are those obsessional Hamlets whose actions are almost completely inhibited by their thoughts. Descartes even based his existence on his thinking: *Cogito ergo sum.* At least he thought this was what he was doing.

This chapter attempts to get a bearing on the problem of doing ethics in our highly scientific and philosophically abstract culture by looking in some depth at the person who must make moral decisions and then act. By looking at the decision-making process, we realize that as important as abstract thought and cognition are, there are other ingredients as well. So completely have thought and action come to be separated in the modern imagination that we have become accustomed to asking the epistemological question "How do we know?" independent of the ethical question "What shall we do?" So thoroughly do we allow ourselves to maintain this split in our minds that often we do not even know who or what we are. We are not only confused but depersonalized by the impersonalization of philosophy and ethics. Thus when we say that ethics involves more than morality—that it is the process of reflecting on values as values are translated into action—we are identifying the person by the actions that person chooses. One is not what one *thinks* but what one *does*—or more precisely, one is *known* by what one does. This is what Hauerwas means when he claims that integrity, not obligation, is the hallmark of moral life. One's wholeness is constituted by one's consistency over a period of time, a lifetime, not in proclaiming what one considers to be virtuous. When Hauerwas faults the standard account of ethics for its attempt to be universal, impersonal, atemporal, and acultural, he is reminding us of what we already know, but are inclined to forget; namely, that ethics is contextual (arising from particular life situations), and it is personal, historical, and cultural. We are inclined to forget this because of the demand that such awareness places on us. We are obligated to follow the admonition "Know thyself" because our sense of identity depends on it, and our moral reputation rests on what we choose to do.

THE CONTEXT OF ETHICAL DECISION MAKING

The critique of the standard account may be summarized and contrasted with its alternative by means of the following chart.

Standard (Regnant) Account	Alternative (Post-Critical) Account
Universal	Contextual
Impersonal	Personal
Atemporal	Historical
Acultural	Cultural
Based on obligation	Based on integrity
Enforced by control, suasion, or sanction	Enforced by willing assent, trust in a convivial order, or community

Each of these features will be examined in some detail in the discussions that follow. We may start by looking at what at first may appear to be a rather mundane clinical situation. If ethics is to be understood as a process of reflecting on the value judgments one makes, that process is very much like clinical judgment for the physician. Does clinical judgment include ethical ingredients even if not recognized as such? Again consider the decision involved in choosing an analgesic:

A 54-year-old engineer is now in his eighth post-op day following abdominal surgery for ulcer repair. While a likable person, this engineer gives the impression of being a chronic complainer, a hypochondriac. And he requests his Demerol for pain always half an hour before it is ordered, once every four hours for pain: His surgeon comes in and talks to him a little bit about it. The surgeon

113

says, "Most of my patients are better by the eighth day. Demerol is a highly addictive medication." After some discussion along these lines, the surgeon says, "Well, I think what I will do is switch you to Talwin for pain. You'll still have your pain medication but with a less addictive drug."[2]

This example has the virtue of illustrating a real conflict that involves more than just technical criteria and facts and that, though of no apparent controversy, is of grave importance to the people involved. The physician might not recognize this as a matter for ethical reflection, thinking it to be merely a matter of clinical judgment. The philosopher/ethicist is quick to spot the value dimensions of this kind of decision and raise in an ethical context the kinds of questions the physician might well also be raising without identifying them as ethical questions *per se*. Is depriving the engineer of the narcotic he requests causing him undue suffering, or conversely, would acceding to his request/demand mean irresponsibility, causing him to become addicted? The matter might in fact become quite controversial if it is recognized that the surgeon is making a judgment about what might be called the engineer's "character," even if that character judgment were camouflaged as a "psychiatric assessment" of addictive potential."

Physicians make numerous such choices every day. When are these decisions to be identified as ethical choices? I submit that a mundane choice is considered an ethical matter when an element of *conflict* is involved. This conflict may be a conflict within oneself: A given individual faces a dilemma between two courses of action, each having some merit; we call this *intrapsychic* conflict. Or the conflict may be between two or more persons committed to different courses of action, which we may call *interpersonal conflict*.

We may hope that when such conflicts arise they can be resolved peacefully, but we can easily imagine that such conflicts might generate friction, heat, antagonism, even anger. Where there is conflict, there is likely to be affect. Ethical discussion often becomes difficult because of the unpleasantness of the affect it generates. Indeed it is such conflict that often occasions ethical reflection. It is a task of ethics to resolve or mediate such conflicts, and many approaches to ethics try to minimize the affect. Objectivity and equanimity are seen as desirable. Analysis of alternatives, it is sometimes suggested, should be rational, cool, dispassionate, and logically rigorous. While this may be desirable, abstract analysis can often miss the point of real conflict and be too remote from the genuine concerns. It is also a task of ethics to identify real concerns, which may have lain dormant because dealing with them would be uncomfortable.

Thus as a starting point and point of orientation when ethical reflection seems to be getting abstract and remote, I often find it useful to ask "Where is the *affect*?" as a way of locating ethical conflict.

At a panel discussion of the Karen Quinlan situation, the problem of when to turn off an artificial respirator was addressed by a physician, a lawyer, and a *philosopher, from the perspectives of their varied disciplines. Each in turn gave a talk outlining the issues from his point of view. The talks were very abstract with qualifications and requalifications about possible definitions of death and how a decision to turn off her respirator might be reached. The comments made had a very detached quality as if the speakers were indifferent to the situation, yet there was an undercurrent of tension, anxiety, perhaps as everyone present imagined being in such a situation and how to deal with it. Where was the affect? Finally a point was raised which seemed initially to be tangential to the substance of the discussion. How much was it costing and who was paying? At that time Karen Quinlan's hospitalization had cost some $130,000 at public expense. Perhaps that should not have mattered, but it did. It was mentioned that Mr. Wrigley, the Chicago chewing gum magnate, had kept his wife alive on a respirator for a number of years at personal expense. The lawyer argued that as long as it was done at personal expense, there was no matter of ethical concern. A political science professor objected very strenuously that who paid was an irrelevant issue, and that there was a real ethical conflict involved. At this point the discussion became very heated and everyone got drawn in. It seemed that one of the key affective issues involved was the issue of money. Who was spending money and how the money was being spent was something about which people had very strong feelings. An issue which started out as a concern with definitions of death, turned out to involve "allocation of scarce resources," distributive justice, and free economy as well.*

These two examples in particular and any of a number of situations we might choose to examine, several of which we will later have occasion to consider, illustrate a problem in ethics, which John Macmurray terms "the crisis of the personal" in philosophy. In the example of choosing an analgesic, we see that it is possible for a person (the physician) to act (to choose an analgesic) without necessarily reflecting on that action. In the extreme of this impersonality the action could become almost reflexive: "I act this way because that's what I always do" or because "that's what is always done, standard procedure." In consideration of the Karen Quinlan panel discussion, we see reflection either with a paucity of affect or an almost uncontrollable excess of affect.* The equivocation in these situations comes from an uncertainty about where to locate the person or how to identify the person. Does one indwell the situation (mind and body, thought and affect)? Or is the person removed from the situation, reflecting on it from the Archimedian point outside the world? Our first instinct might say both or either, so accustomed have we become to moving back and forth by acts of mental distancing. Because of this acquired ability, we should take a closer look at what is meant by the personal.

---

*The task of the ethicist is in at least one very important regard similar to that of the psychotherapist or psychoanalyst: in the attempt to achieve the right titration of affect so that learning about human experience may take place. When confronted by a hyper-rational elaboration of detail and an isolation of affect, it is necessary to raise the titer of emotion. When confronted with hysterical overemotionality, the task is to lower the level of affect, so that reason may have an opportunity.

PERSONHOOD

What is a self, a person? We may easily be misled if we follow a philosophy based on understanding the physical universe; we are not merely atoms, which mean nothing more to one another than an occasional bump in a vast emptiness. The word "person" was in its earliest forms the Latin "persona," the mask worn by actors in a drama. The linguistic clue suggests an awareness of the equivocation in selfhood, for the mask that one presented publicly was not necessarily the private self. Indeed there is the inherent possibility for self-deception in assuming a public role to disclose one's conscious intentions, for if one holds up a mirror to oneself, it may be the mask that looks back.

But the mask cannot be worn at all times, so one must look again and again to know a self. A self is dynamic, not static; it changes and develops over time. This is what it means to have a history and to live and act in history. When one is identified by a variety of the predicates that one might choose, for example, I am a . . . carpenter, father, Christian, male, diabetic, Democrat, teenager, or whatever, these are but partial identities, chosen for the sake of expediency to attempt to convey something more complex than language can easily disclose. One's self must encompass all that one is and has been, a totality of life history and its memories, not all of which are accessible to conscious memory at any one time, many of which one might wish to delete and may do so by selective amnesia. Somerset Maugham recognized this when he said:

> What makes old age hard to bear is not a failing of one's faculties, mental and physical, but the burden of one's memories.[3]

The view of history Maugham is expressing is not the one that is so often held, the chronicle of time or march of events, but a very personal view, one that Merleau-Ponty has called "temporal thickness."[4] History is not just the public and recorded events, but each person has a unique history of his or her own. Furthermore, it must be emphatically emphasized that this history extends back to childhood and to birth, though the earliest memories may be obliterated. It is important to keep this point in mind as we reconsider the meaning of the personal, the historical, the temporal, and the cultural in relation to ethics, for the early antecedents of rationality have some forms that are very different from the adult thought processes that are usually meant when one refers to "rationality." History is not just the chronicle of events of successive generations of rational adults, as we might find in the textbooks, but each person starts as an irrational child and carries into adult life the childhood antecedents of prerational thought, what psychiatrists call "primary process" thinking.

According to Piaget's studies of cognitive development, there is a disjunc-

116

tion in cognitive processes that occurs around the onset of adolescence. At this time,

> the child achieves the [Cartesian] *cogito* and reaches the truths of rationalism. At this stage . . . he discovers himself both as a point of view on the world and also as called upon to transcend that point of view and to construct an objectivity at the level of judgment.[5]

The *cogito* thus becomes the child's passport to adult society. As he learns the rules of his culture by living them, he develops a critical sense. Thus supported by the norms of his group, he acquires a sure standard for judgment. And as a self-assured judge, he of course is less vulnerable himself. Yet even while recognizing this developmental transition, Piaget brings to the child a mature outlook, as if the thoughts of the adult were self-sufficient and devoid of all contradiction. In reality, as Merleau-Ponty reminds us,

> it must be the case that the child's outlook is in some way vindicated against the adult's and against Piaget, and that the unsophisticated thinking of our earliest years remains as an indispensable acquisition underlying that of maturity.[6]

The study of philosophy is an undertaking of the rational mind. As a branch of philosophy, ethics is a rational undertaking. Yet people do not always behave in rational ways, and ethics must account for this irrationality in human behavior. As a way of getting beyond the limitations imposed on ethics by an impersonal view of objectivity, I am proposing that a look at the childhood antecedents of rationality is useful. There are several avenues to this understanding, which converge to broaden the conception of what ethical reflection may be able to accomplish. One is psychoanalysis, which emerged historically at the time when critical thought was gaining its greatest incisiveness, indeed at a time when logical positivism was emerging in Vienna and elsewhere. Another useful approach is the ethical revisions offered by such philosophers as Edmund Pincoffs or Stanley Hauerwas, who suggest that narrative accounts of the life stories of those involved in making decisions offer clues to the ethical issues at stake. John Macmurray offers a critique of traditional philosophy, which suggests possible reorientations, and Michael Polanyi's epistemology similarly offers new possibilities for ethics. As we better appreciate the limitations objectivist epistemology poses for ethics, we are in a better position to consider alternatives that may be more productive.

THE CRISIS OF THE PERSONAL

John Macmurray in his Gifford Lectures of 1953, given under the title "The Form of the Personal" and published under the title *The Self as Agent*, identifies what he calls "the crisis of the personal." Macmurray is concerned that modern philosophy has led to a situation in which man is seen impersonally, thus impeding the possibility of accounting for man in relation either to other persons or to God ("always an 'I,' never a 'Thou'"). He levels two charges against philosophy: (1) that it is merely theoretical and (2) that it is egocentric. Of the first charge he notes:

> Philosophy aims at a complete rationality. But the rationality of our conclusions does not depend alone upon the correctness of our thinking. It depends even more upon the propriety of the questions with which we concern ourselves. The primary and the critical task is the discovery of the problem. If we ask the wrong question the logical correctness of our answer is of little consequence.[7]

He further notes that "Common tradition conceives the philosopher as a man of a balanced temper, who meets fortune or disaster with equanimity."[8] The theory with which philosophy deals must be rooted in the practical questions which man experiences or it risks being trivial or misleading.

Of the second charge, that modern philosophy is egocentric, he notes that "It takes the Self as its starting-point, and not God, or the world or the community; and that the Self is seen as an individual in isolation, withdrawn from active relations with other selves." About this solipsistic outlook much more is said in the following chapter, but for the time being we must note the distortion in the notion of a self, of a person.

Macmurray proposes to redress this imbalance by transferring the center of gravity in philosophy from thought to action. It is in this sense that he defines the self as an agent and attempts to substitute the "I do" for the "I think" as the defining characteristic of personhood.

Considerations of thought are static; they do not move. Considerations of action are dynamic, and we may inquire into the forces that cause motion. In so doing we rely metaphorically on the mechanical images of physical forces moving bodies through space and time in order to grasp something of mental life and experience, which so elude our understanding. Gilbert Ryle speaks of the mind as the "ghost in the machine"[9] as a way of helping us through the familiar layers of philosophical thought to an understanding of mental life. This metaphor reflects the habitual ways we have come to understand ourselves.

THE MORAL SELF

Freud similarly relied on mechanical metaphors in his attempt to elucidate the unconscious realms of mental life. When he spoke of psychodynamics, he was casting in scientific language the mythologies of the ages and returning us to the histories of persons. To understand ethics—that is, to understand persons who act and make decisions in history—it is necessary to understand the forces that move people. We do not really want a passionless philosophy, but rather want to understand the emotions that underlie philosophical deliberation, even though we constantly fear that sanctioning the recognition of these forces will unleash uncivilized demons that might better remain contained.[10]

What forces underlie morality? What emotions or affects provide the dynamos that move people to action? By asking these questions, what are we able to accomplish that a merely theoretical and egocentric philosophy cannot accomplish? What is the self that acts in history and how does knowledge of this self, ourself, help us in making decisions in relation both to the situations in which we find ourselves and also to those principles that we are able abstractly to adduce?

This nest of questions is complex. They might correctly be answered by saying that all emotions in one way or another at some time or another influence the way people act. Therefore, we must quickly limit our focus to specific emotions and situations by way of example or remain forever on a theoretical level. The clues from the psychoanalytic study of problems in self-esteem and the devices by which a person regulates self-esteem through morality therefore are illuminating.

The psychoanalytic study of the self derives from Freud's early observations in "On Narcissism: An Introduction,"[11] in which he introduced the concept of the ego ideal, also sometimes referred to as the ideal self, which later gave origin to the concept of the superego in Freud's topographic (id, ego, superego) theory of personality development.[12] The term "narcissism" is derived from clinical description and was chosen by Paul Nacke in 1899 to denote the attitude of a person who treats his own body in the same way in which the body of a sexual object is ordinarily treated. Freud at that time was developing his libido theory, which derived support from the studies of children and from primitive peoples. "Totem and Taboo"[13] preceded Freud's work on narcissism, and Jung's departure from psychoanalysis occurred about this time in protest of Freud's insistence on infantile sexuality. Autoeroticism was clearly evident in the normal development of children, a pleasurable "instinct" from the start, but the ego, that mental agency that mediates and regulates the impulses, had to be developed over time.

The study of primitive cultures' abhorrence of incest and the function of taboos against it demonstrated the dynamic forces that enabled these forces to be suppressed, and the unacceptable (hostile, murderous, even sexual) impulses of children in civilized Vienna followed the patterns of the primitives. Libidinal instinctual impulses undergo pathological repression if they come into conflict with the person's cultural and ethical ideas. The formation of an ego ideal and later a superego are the devices by which the young child can learn to live harmoniously in a family and in a culture. They are pleasurable deceptions, which the child can unconsciously maintain while the ego gradually learns how to cope with reality.

Freud declared the ego ideal to be the "heir of the original narcissism"[14] and Hartman and Lowenstein say, "the ego ideal can be considered a rescue operation for narcissism."[15] In other words the ego ideal is born of an effort to restore the lost pleasures of the symbiosis with an all-giving mother. In this blissful state the human infant lies securely at the center of his universe. His every need is met by a mother (or sometimes another) who needs him almost as much as he needs her. He is omnipotent. If he is hungry or in some other way uncomfortable, he cries, and mother comes to meet the need. This state is referred to as primary narcissism, but it is a precarious condition.

The enemy of primary narcissism is the reality principle. The symbiosis is ruptured too soon after the infant is expelled from the womb. He is hungry and cries, but the mother does not immediately appear. The universe is not perfect as he had imagined, and it is not under his control. The result is rage, possibly despair if he is abandoned or if his mother is not dependable. The original sense of omnipotence has received the first of many "narcissistic injuries." Reality has entered in.

The infant copes with this intrusion by shifting focus to an idealized parent; it is not he but the parent that is perfect. As the infant's physical and mental abilities, particularly locomotion, develop, it is less necessary to be completely dependent on the mother, and the infant becomes aware of his separateness from her. The small, helpless infant forms an ideal of what he would like to be; that is, omnipotent like the parents. But even under the best of circumstances, the idealized parents prove fallible, incapable of providing the total gratification remembered from earliest infancy, and the infant develops a new and better possibility for the self, the ego ideal. The love that was originally invested in the self and then in the idealized parent is now invested in the ideal self that he desires to become. This state is called secondary narcissism. Freud observed that man creates ideals for himself to restore the lost narcissism of childhood, to restore that state of contentment in which one's needs are passively met. It is the ego ideal, Freud claims, "by which the ego measures itself, towards which it strives, and whose demands for ever-increasing perfection it is always striving to fulfill."[16] But the grandiose aspirations for perfection in reality can never be fulfilled. A person's self-esteem is determined by the distance between his actual self—his strengths, talents, abilities, and accomplishments—and his ego ideal.

The superego, thought by many psychoanalysts to be distinct from the ego ideal, is a developmentally later acquisition. In contrast to the ego ideal, which lures the person on to higher and often impossible standards of perfection, the superego is restrictive. It is the superego that is the internalized representation of the parents and of the culture's standards for conduct. The superego is the unconscious conscience that criticizes the id impulses and keeps the ego in line. Instinctual gratification (whether sexual or aggressive) is renounced either out of fear of loss of love by the ego ideal or by fear of punishment by the superego. This is why Freud suggests in "Civilization and its Discontents"[17] that neurosis is the price we must pay for the harmony of civilized culture, a verdict that is only reluctantly accepted.

Earlier I contrasted upward and downward perspectives on tasks of ethics. Considered not only in terms of the function of ethical theory but also of the development of an individual, it may now be said that ethics in the upward perspective functions by means of the ego ideal, and ethics in the downward perspective functions by means of the superego. One is beckoned upward by the highest standards of moral perfection, but restricted from falling below certain minimal standards by means of superego strictures, if internalized, and by the possibility of external punishment if necessary. Teleological ethical theories appeal to goals that all might be expected to hold. Deontological ethical theories set standards by which one may know what limitations are expected. Earlier I criticized the standard account of ethics as being inadequate because it attempts to be universal, impersonal, acultural, and ahistorical. I now add that teleological and deontological accounts are both inadequate. They fail us not only because they are too abstract but also because they rest on immature developmental forms, the ego ideal and the superego. With this said, we may now explore in greater depth the affects associated with the ego ideal and the superego and why they are inadequate as a basis for morality.

SHAME AND GUILT AS REGULATORS OF MORALITY

Morality in any given culture is enforced by the affects of shame and guilt. Shame is the primary affect that mediates the functioning of the ego ideal in a given person, and guilt is the affect by which the superego exerts its force. *Shame* consists of feelings of inferiority, humiliation, embarrassment, inadequacy, incompetence, weakness, dishonor, disgrace, "loss of face"; the feeling of being vulnerable to or actually experiencing ridicule, contempt, insult, derision, scorn, rejection, or other "narcissistic wounds"; and the feeling of not being able to take care of oneself and of being dependent on others. Jealousy and envy are members of this family of feelings. *Guilt* refers to the feeling of having committed a sin, a crime, an evil, or an injustice; the feeling of culpability; the feeling of obligation; the feeling of being dangerous or harmful to others; and the feeling of needing expiation and deserving punishment.

James Gilligan in a very provocative analysis, "Beyond Morality: Psychoanalytic Reflections on Shame, Guilt, and Love," sees morality as a "force antagonistic to love, a force causing illness and death—neurosis and psychosis, homicide and suicide." He views morality as a "necessary but immature stage of affective and cognitive development, so that fixation at the moral stage represents developmental retardation, or immaturity, and regression to it represents psychopathology, or neurosis.[18] He claims that morality is dead, that it killed itself. Citing the self-criticism moral philosophy has subjected

121

itself to over the past two centuries (for example, Hume, Kant, Nietzsche, and Wittgenstein), he believes that the only knowledge possible is of scientific facts, not moral value.

As evidence for this, he draws on demonstrations of the effects of shame and guilt in various cultures. An example of a pure shame culture is the Kwakiutl Indians of Vancouver Island, described by Ruth Benedict:

> Behavior ... was dominated at every point by the need to demonstrate the greatness of the individual and the inferiority of his rivals. It was carried out with uncensored self-glorification and with gibes and insults poured upon the opponents. ... The Kwakiutl stressed equally the fear of ridicule, and the interpretation of experience in terms of insults. They recognized only one gamut of emotion, that which swings between victory and shame.[19]

An example of a pure guilt culture is the Hutterites, a Protestant sect scattered through the northern Middle West and southern Canada on communal farms and colonies, where they consciously attempt to adhere strictly and literally to the ethic of the New Testament. They are described by Kaplan and Plaut:

> Religion is the major cohesive force in this folk culture. The Hutterites consider themselves to ... live the only true form of Christianity, one which entails communal sharing of property and cooperative production and distribution of goods. The values of brotherliness, self-renunciation and passivity in the face of aggression are emphasized. The Hutterites speak often of their past martyrs and of their willingness to suffer for their faith at the present time.[20]

In these extreme forms shame cultures display a maximum of hostility toward others in order to maintain a maximum of love for the self; the guilt cultures display a minimum of love for the self in order to check hostility toward others and maintain nonviolence and pacifism.

I am in fundamental agreement with Gilligan's contention that morality can be a destructive force if it excessively relies on shame and guilt. I disagree that morality must necessarily be destructive, however. Considered in historical perspective—that is, in developmental perspective—morality serves the growing person well by providing an orientation to one's culture and to those others with whom one lives. Morality also provides a sense of identity, that understanding of self by which one lives, and by which one is known to others. This sense of agency, however, is achieved gradually over time and emerges from the immature forms of the ego ideal and superego. The mature sense of agency carries with it the sense of competence, empowerment, potency, internal force, confidence in initiating change or control, and a realistic appraisal of what it may be possible and appropriate to accomplish.[21] The mature agent has more or less successfully resolved his narcissism: His expectations for himself and his (ego) ideals are more or less in line with his abilities, and his goals, though perhaps ambitious, are neither grandiose nor represent a striving for omnipotent perfection. Given the vicissitudes of human development, this state of mature agency is not usually achieved. Even when it is achieved, it is in precarious balance with those stresses in life that would precipitate helplessness and dependency: the various life crises, loss of loved ones, aging, and especially the loss of one's health through unexpected illness. These stresses may bring forth a yearning for an ideal world and a return to a state of blissful dependency, and that yearning may include the idealized wish for the physician to be an omnipotent god, a wish the physician may be seduced into sharing. Such dependency, however, engenders much ambivalence, especially in a culture that so values independence, self-reliance, and autonomy. When reflecting ethically on the possibilities for such an ideal world, we must be mindful of our own narcissistic temptations and keep reality firmly in view.

There is nothing wrong with maintaining perfectionistic ideals unless they are used destructively to clobber mortal humans who cannot live up to their standards. It is these immature and grandiose forms of morality that can be destructive.

THE PROBLEM OF THE MORAL INVERSION

We must now turn to a consideration of the destructive force of *excesses* of morality and the demand for moral perfection. In the appendix to this chapter, some of the positive, life-sustaining characteristics of morality are further considered. The thesis advanced here is that values form the core of the identity of a person and thus regulate self-esteem. If viewed from the perspective of the regnant epistemology, which defines a person in terms of thought instead of action, morality becomes a destructive force. In its abstract forms, morality insists on moral perfection, which no person can achieve. Gilligan is right insofar as he views morality in the context of the standard epistemological accounts of morality. Morality has killed itself, or rather, it has failed to give an adequate account of itself. However, we may carry Gilligan's use of the psychoanalytic approach and Polanyi's use of the post-critical approach beyond the limitations of the standard/regnant account to demonstrate that love or trust as the most fundamental and earliest developmental issue is the correct basis for morality, not shame or guilt, which represent pathological aberrations if not properly resolved. This stands in staunch opposition to the view that holds (solipsistically) that the autonomy of persons is the basis for ethics. Such a view cannot be true because persons are in no real way autonomous; they exist in relationship with others, whom they may or may not trust, but on whom they are unquestionably dependent and interdependent. Descartes's dualistic philosophy bases knowledge on doubt rather than belief (trust) because, I believe, of his own insecurity in trusting an insecurity that touches all of us fundamentally because of the developmental traumas we must face in early childhood. Polanyi corrects the Cartesian mistake by reminding us that we never have been able to base knowledge on doubt; rather, knowledge rests, now in modern science as it always has, on a fiduciary enterprise of a community of knowers rather than on the isolated efforts of individuals who bear no relationship to one another.

The epistemological work of Michael Polanyi is useful as a counterbalance to such excesses.[22] I believe it may be shown that ethics follows quite legitimately from epistemology by rooting one's knowledge in the commitments one holds. Himself a scientist (initially trained as a physician), Polanyi took exception to the objectivist view of science by demonstrating the "tacit dimension" of knowing in the process of scientific discovery. His post-critical epistemology seeks unification of the sciences and the humanities by stressing the role of the knower in the knowing. Only in a culture admitting to a scientist-humanist dichotomy could there be such ambiguity about the role of the physician.

The moral inversion is a phenomenon in which moral passions are repudiated in the face of strict scientific objectivity. What happens in the repudiation is often a reversal or inversion in which quite immoral ends are justified scientifically. Polanyi sees the moral inversion as being derived from conflicting aims of our knowledge. He sees two conflicting ideals of our age (moral passions and intellectual skepticism) "locked in a curious struggle in which they may combine and reinforce each other."[23]

The moral inversion comes about when an individual feels unable to meet the absolute ideals of moral perfection. Such an individual imbued with the demands of critical objectivity sees such moral perfectionism as hypocritical (literally less than critical) and repudiates it in the name of something honest, authentic, or real. Often this may be some social cause that derives its merit from simplification of a complex situation, or it may be an utterly gratuitous act, which has nothing more to commend it than the fact that it is indeed chosen.

The example of the 23-year-old mother whose lawyers opposed involuntary commitment may be understood as a moral inversion. Rigid adherence to the principle of liberty, which is good for the preservation of a free society, is cruelly immoral for the woman who ended up dead.

Existentialist literature offers numerous examples in which gratuitous acts affirm the reality of the individual who would otherwise feel dehumanized in an objectivist world. Dostoevsky's Raskolnikov in *Crime and Punishment* is a prime example. By murdering the old woman *for no reason* he can order his otherwise senseless existence. Andre Gide's Lafcadio similarly vindicates himself by pushing a man off the train. The moral inversion is so prevalent in American cinema as to be commonplace. The cinema extols its antiheros; the good guys are the bad guys, who are admired for their audacious defiance of hypocritical social convention. Butch Cassidy and the Sundance Kid rob bad banks for the sheer fun of it. Bonnie and Clyde perform the same crimes to overcome impotence. In *A Clockwork Orange*, an honestly self-serving psychopath is attractive when compared to the behavior modifiers for whom behavioral ends justify cruel means.

Polanyi's key example is what he calls the "dynamo-objective coupling" of Soviet Marxism, which he uses to illustrate the proximity of morality to politics and the close reciprocal workings of moral passions with an objective view of reality.[24] In the dynamo-objective coupling, alleged scientific assertions, which are accepted as such because they satisfy moral passions, will excite these passions still further and thus lend increased conviction to the scientific affirmations in question, and so on. Moreover, such a dynamo-objective coupling is also potent in its own defense; any criticism of its scientific part is rebutted by the moral passions behind it, while any moral objections are coldly brushed aside by involving the inexorable verdict of its scientific finding.

In the Marxist example, one sees a coupling between the utopian ideals—liberty, justice, and brotherhood—and their translation into an objectivistic view of the social order, namely, dialectic materialism. By covering moral passions with a scientific disguise, moral sentiments are protected against depreciation as mere emotionalism. They acquire instead a sense of scientific certainty. On the other hand, material ends are impregnated with the fervor of moral passions.

In modern psychiatry and behavioral science, examples of the moral inversion are also quite common. The disciplines—to the extent that they remain bound by the tenets of positivism—disclaim any moral intentions. Yet the vast enterprises of psychiatry, psychoanalysis, behavior modification, and counseling proceed according to value judgments, with the metaphors health or illness or the measurements normal or abnormal surviving as surrogates for the moral terms good or bad (valued or disvalued).

Thus the antipsychiatrists have a point in their criticism of psychiatry for its failure to give attention to moral values. The antipsychiatry movement is an example of a critical approach to ethics—the criticism of an articulated or implied moral position. Psychiatry as a profession is vulnerable to this criticism because its ethics are implicit, tacit, sometimes unconscious, and usually tied up with a social consensus of how much deviant behavior a given community will tolerate. Civil rights, human rights, and personal rights are often the vehicles for calling attention to such value controversies. The psychiatric detention of political dissenters by the Soviets is an extreme example of the interconnections between shared social beliefs and psychiatric practice.

If one believes Marxist doctrine, that is, believes it to be a correct explanation of reality, then someone who dissents from that doctrine could legitimately be considered to be out of touch with reality. Conversely, a psychiatrist recognizing the realities of harsh political treatment could argue that psychiatric detention is a more humane compromise.

These arguments confuse concepts of rights (morality) with concepts of reality (facts). The Soviet system probably has more in common epistemolo-gically with American psychiatry than advocates of human rights would care to acknowledge, even though the moral outlooks are very different. Both are thoroughly modern in their camouflaging of social beliefs with scientifically objective facts. Neither system attempts a systematic articulation of moral principles. The moral passions of the antipsychiatrists, however, become inverted in a passionate therapeutic nihilism that would destroy anything short of perfection and along with it the possibility of genuine moral enrichment.

The Marxist example is a fruitful one for Western medicine because one of the focal conflicts is that between the individualism of medicine and the socialism of the economic system that supports it. As high-technology medicine becomes more and more expensive, we are increasingly forced to look at the tension between the needs of the individual and the cost to society. We are forced to ask tough questions about allocation of resources and about individual and societal responsibility. Witness the millions of dollars spent on Medicare for renal dialysis and the scant funding for public health, which might shift some of the cost and responsibility from treatment of debilitating illness to its prevention.

CONCLUSIONS

Earlier the question of a methodology for ethics was raised, suggesting that the force of the critical tradition tends to depersonalize ethics by abstracting thought from action. Generally speaking, ethical issues are raised around points of conflict—either an *interpersonal conflict* in which two or more people are committed to different courses of action or an *intrapsychic conflict* in which a given person may see compelling reasons for conflicting decisions. Modern medicine seldom offers us the clear-cut alternatives that could neatly be dissected as *either* good *or* bad, or *either* right *or* wrong. Instead, we are offered complex situations in which any course of action compromises certain ethical principles, and few decisions can be made with more certainty than ambiguity.

We are a very narcissistic society. By this I mean not so much that we are self-indulgent, although this may be the case, but that we are ruthless in the pursuit of our ideals. Often, ethical norms serve as impossible ideals, which we should strive toward but can never live up to. If we recognize these ideals as just that, then I believe we have set the stage for a humanistic approach to medicine. If we try to translate these ideals into imperatives, we run the risk of further moral inversions as the already grandiose expectations of medicine become inflated even further, and we begin to think perfectionistically rather than realistically.

If we can succeed in establishing ideals that are sufficiently general as to be applicable in most situations, we can save wear and tear on our consciences, but this generalizing risks being rigid and unresponsive to human needs. Indeed, I suspect that much of the social criticism of medicine as mechanistic and dehumanizing actually stems ironically from medicine's unyielding idealism.

A humanistic approach to medicine must recognize and be responsive to the diverse and often contrary individuality of our human lot; few rigid principles are sufficiently flexible to account for such diversity. Humanistic medicine also must recognize and tolerate the humanity of physicians. Grandiose perfectionism often results in stereotyped idealism rather than mutual respect and further contributes to the unrealistic ideal of physician omniscience and omnipotence.

CHAPTER 9

THE IMPEACHMENT OF
ALTRUISM

PHYSICIANS HAVE traditionally oriented themselves by an ideal of service that is often called "altruistic." Ideals of course are goals and not realities. But it nonetheless comes as a rude shock to many physicians to realize that their ideals are no longer credible. The problem is not just that physicians— individually or collectively—have failed to live up to the service ideal, but that any ideals ring hollow in a hard-nosed and pragmatic age.

Altruism is an endangered species. It is on the verge of extinction. We may not have seen the end of altruism, of concern for the well-being of others, and of some of the nobler forms of human conduct, but the word "altruism" has lost its usefulness. It has lost its ability to serve as a vehicle of moral inspiration. Altruism, however, is in good company. Other words of our moral vocabulary have similarly been rendered antique. Sin, restitution, virtue, chastity, and guilt (except in a therapeutic sense) have all but disappeared from ordinary language, leaving us handicapped in talking about moral issues.

Narcissism, on the other hand, is just coming into its own. The word "narcissism," which is in many ways the opposite of altruism, serves an increasingly useful function in calling attention to the shape and contours of the culture in which we live. Christopher Lasch suggests that we have become a "Culture of Narcissism."[1] Does this mean that selfishness, or narcissism, has gained the upper hand over selflessness, or altruism? I think not. What I am suggesting instead is that in contemporary culture the ideals suggested by the word "altruism" are so difficult to fulfill that they seem incredible, literally, not believable. Anyone professing to be altruistic is suspect, whereas anyone professing self-interest is hailed as honest if not admirable.

The word "altruism" is only about 125 years old, having been coined by Auguste Comte,[2] who also gave us "sociology." But the idea of sacrificing oneself for the welfare of others goes back to the foundations of our philosophical heritage, to Plato and to early Christian traditions. Western thought is so habitually ethical that most people never suspect that it could be otherwise.

In the late nineteenth century, at a time when the AMA was trying to consolidate a professional identity based on scientific medicine and an ethic of service, the United States offered a fertile ground for the concept of altruism according to an account offered by Louis Budd.[3] It was a time of laissez-faire capitalism and the heyday of the "work ethic." A candid look at the ethics of the time might suggest a world dominated by self-interest, by greed, and by opportunism. Yet it was also a time of intense religiosity in which ethical justification was sought for human conduct, perhaps defensively and rationalistically. Altruism provided a rallying point for reforms that collided head-on with the premise of man's selfishness. It was celebrated in magazines, novels, and altrurian societies of a utopian sort.

Nineteenth-century altruists preached that progress was the object of nature and that altruism was the object of progress. They extolled altruism as the instinct that had equalized and thus healthily intensified the competitive struggle, making, in other words, for more of a fair fight. This was a time of Social Darwinism, in which "the survival of the fittest" provided natural justification for those who got ahead at the expense of others. "Nature, red in tooth and claw"—this not only explained the origin of species but also provided a justification for the accumulation of capital.

It may be difficult to imagine what it was like to live in those turbulent times and to see man taken from his special place in nature and tossed among the brutes by the theory of evolution. Altruism may have served to preserve a sense of the nobility of our own species, but not all views of human nature are optimistic. Consider this analysis of "The Antisocial Contract."

> The evolution of society fits the Darwinian paradigm in its most individualistic form. Nothing in it cries out to be explained otherwise. The economy of nature is competitive from beginning to end. . . . No hint of genuine charity ameliorates our vision of society, once sentimentalism has been laid aside. What passes for cooperation turns out to be a mixture of opportunism and exploitation. . . . Where it is in his own interest, every organism may reasonably be expected to aid his fellows. Where he has no alternative he submits to the yoke of communal servitude. Yet given a full chance to act in his own interest, nothing but expediency will restrain him from brutalizing, from maiming, from murdering—his brother, his mate, his parent, or his child. Scratch an "altruist," and watch a "hypocrite" bleed.[4]

Altruism is hardly credible as a pure explanation of human motivation, given what we now know about human dynamics. It now seems obvious that the altruists of the 1890s saw personality too unitarily, as either benign or vicious. We now recognize that kindly (or hostile) behavior can have mixed, ambivalent motives that can also differ from one person to the next and from time to time in a given individual. Recall that Freud published *The Interpretation of Dreams* in 1900, and it is only in this century that depth psychology has become part of our intellectual baggage and habitual way of looking at things. Even today there is great resistance to looking too deeply.

The altruists of the nineteenth century underestimated the strength of the ego's self-serving drive and thought they could soothe it away. They had limitless faith in moral suasion. Today the magnitude and the velocity of the social change make gentle moral appeals sound quixotic, while the anonymity of urbanism mocks any dream of promoting altruism by personal example.

In spite of all its shortcomings, altruism has an amazing buoyancy. Moral inclinations, of course, live on even though moral perfection is not possible. After years of dormancy, the word "altruism" is now making a comeback. The new altruism, however, has a special meaning that is potentially a source of confusion. For biologists, and particularly for the new discipline known as sociobiology,[5] altruism involved self-sacrifice for the welfare of a group of genetically related others. The biological implications of altruism are long term and concerned with behavior that would likely continue the species, whereas the familiar use of altruism refers to unselfish regard for the welfare of others in a day-to-day manner. The Good Samaritan is an example of an old-fashioned altruist. His actions were not in response to social pressures or moral obligations; he acted gratuitously and in a way that was costly to himself. These are tenets of altruism as we generally think of it. The behavior of the social insects ants, bees, and termites are examples of the new altruism. The sacrifices of the worker bees ensure the furtherance of the species by enabling the queen to reproduce. Thus, it becomes necessary to distinguish the new altruism, which refers to species-maintaining behavior, from traditional altruism, which refers to individual nonreciprocal giving.

For our purposes in understanding the dynamics of moral life, we could largely ignore the specialized use of the term "altruism" by the sociobiologists except for the irresistible temptation to draw parallels between the evolution of behavior of the social insects and that of humans. Admittedly one can see analogies between army ants and human beings. Both have an urban social order, stored foodstuffs, full-time division of labor, and apartment living. It is not difficult to see the ways in which self-sacrifice in social insects serves to further reproduction of genes. The confusion arises when too facile an analogy is drawn with human behavior. We forget what we are trying to understand when we use the two kinds of altruism interchangeably. Also, animal traits sometimes are given familiar names like coyness, spite, jealousy, selfishness, deceitfulness, greediness, and cooperativeness, with the explicit assumption that specific genes determine these traits. Polanyi calls this mental process a pseudo-substitution.[6]

The new discipline of sociobiology and in particular the issue of the genetics of altruism are causing a lot of debate these days. It may be useful to focus on social evolution to understand the place of moral tradition in contemporary society. As I suggested earlier, we have become almost embarrassed to speak of moral tradition, although the inclination to morality is not quite so alien to us. We are asked by the sociobiologists to believe that the presence of altruism in insects and other nonhumans in some way provides justification—indeed scientific justification—for altruistic behavior that seems to have lost its moral compulsion.

I believe the analogies between the two kinds of altruism (let's now call them moral altruism and behavioral altruism) are too tenuous to use the terms interchangeably. Furthermore, the so-called scientific justification of altruism on genetic-adaptive grounds obscures the essential moral issues, which deserve consideration in their own right. Nonetheless, the interesting development of sociobiology and the sketching of its implications for moral tradition tell us something very important about moral life in an age that is both habitually ethical and habitually scientific in its manner of thinking.

Let me give what I believe to be an important example of the issues at stake. Donald Campbell argues in a major paper entitled "On the Conflicts Between Biological and Social Evolution and Between Psychology and Moral Tradition" that "present-day psychology and psychiatry in all their major forms are more hostile to the inhibitory messages of traditional religious moralizing than is scientifically justified."[7] He further argues on the basis of the genetics of altruism that basic biological human nature is in agreement with traditional religious moral teachings. He notes that "the religions of all ancient urban civilization (as independently developed in China, India, Mesopotamia, Egypt, Mexico, and Peru) taught that many aspects of human nature need to be curbed if optimal coordination is to be achieved; for example, selfishness, pride, greed, dishonesty, covetousness, cowardice, lust, wrath."[8] According to Campbell, "Psychology and psychiatry not only describe man as selfishly motivated, but implicitly or explicitly teach that he ought to be so. They tend to see repression and inhibition of individual impulse as undesirable, and see all guilt as a dysfunctional neurotic blight created by cruel child rearing and a needlessly repressive society. They further recommend that we accept our biological and psychological impulses as good and seek pleasure rather than enchain ourselves with duty."[9]

Campbell's characterization of psychology and psychiatry is obviously overly general, but he does make an important point. It is in fact a point made by Karl Menninger in his book, *Whatever Became of Sin?*[10] Menninger notes that sin—that is, the *concept* of sin—seems to have disappeared from our society, having been translated into other considerations, such as a new social morality, crime, symptoms, or collective irresponsibility. But it is no longer used to mean the abdication of personal responsibility. This was the point I started out with, and this is a point that Campbell also makes in reference to Menninger:

> I am indeed asserting a social functionality and psychological validity to con-
> cepts such as temptation and original sin due to human carnal, animal nature.
> This orientation makes me sympathetic to psychotherapists such as Mowrer and
> Menninger who have come to regard much human sin with an almost traditional
> disapproval, and who are recommending that guilt feelings often should be
> cured by confession, expiation, restitution, and cessation of guilt-producing
> behavior, rather than by always removing the demands of conscience, interpret-
> ing away feelings of guilt as neurotic symptoms. I can only hope that by raising

THE IMPEACHMENT OF ALTRUISM

this conclusion in the context of modern scientific concerns about the problems of complex social coordination and the population genetics of altruistic traits, I can make the point more convincing to psychologists and psychiatrists than Mowrer and Menninger have been able to do.[11]

I would suggest instead that we need to reaccredit our moral vocabulary and acknowledge the place of virtue and character in our lives. We need to speak about moral issues as moral issues. This enterprise may require some hard self-scrutiny. What are the resistances within ourselves to making value judgments and acknowledging them publicly?

A major resistance to self-scrutiny and to addressing moral issues is our narcissism or sense of self. Narcissism is derived metaphorically from the Greek hero Narcissus, who was a lad so beautiful that all the lovely maidens fell in love with him, but he was unable to care for any of them and left them broken-hearted. Finally seeing his image reflected in a pond, he knew what they longed for and fell in love with his own image. Narcissus's fate varies in different versions of the story. His outcome is pathetic. Some say he drowned trying to merge with his image. Others say he pined away at the pool being unable to separate from his image.[12] In any case, he left us with the flower bearing his name and the psychological condition of self-love.

The major problem in the narcissistic syndrome is uncertainty, not confidence. For the narcissistic personality, uncertainty about one's self, one's identity, requires a mirroring reassurance from others that one is okay. The experience is derived from earliest infancy, and in adolescence, if all goes well, one may achieve a sense of stability. If, however, a culture fails to provide a mirror of stability by which one can define oneself, the resolution of a sense of self may not occur until much later in life, if at all. It is often suggested that our own culture is such a culture of narcissism[13] and fails to provide clear-cut standards and ideals by which people may identify themselves and establish a sense of selfhood. The camouflaging of moral issues in scientific or value-neutral garb is one example of this failure.

In a pluralistic and rapidly changing culture, an adolescent may fail to get unambiguous messages about socially acceptable values and expectations. Even so, the nuclear family or even single parents may still serve such a function, although this is increasingly difficult given the erosion of cultural support for the family. In the absence of stable families, family substitutes often emerge. The altrurian societies of the nineteenth century may have served as such value-defining groups. On the contemporary scene we witness the emergence of family-like cults, such as the Charles Manson "family" and the Jim Jones cult in Guyana. Whereas the nineteenth-century communities were defined by positive or prosocial values, we are now seeing the institutionalization of antisocial or demonic values. This inversion of morality can only be seen as demonstrating the urgent need for self-definition when the self is confronted with total isolation and alienation.

133

Narcissism may be seen negatively as resulting from loss of inhibitory moral traditions resulting in unbridled grandiosity and self-interest. But the adaptive advantages must also be noted. In a complex urban world where individualism counts for very little, any attempt to define the self, however grandiose, may serve the individual well as a defense against the worse fate of anonymity and dissolution. Reason itself may be understood as an ego ideal—never quite attainable and only approximated at the cost of isolation from the self; that is, from the feelings and passions that are as much a part of human actions as are abstract ideas, although never completely explicit or conscious. Ethics may get swept up in a ruthless perfectionism, treating abstract ideals as moral imperatives rather than recognizing the inherent limitations in every human endeavor.

During the adolescent period, if all goes well, the moral personality emerges with its emphasis on personal dignity and self-esteem rather than superego dependency and instinctual gratification. The ego ideal in many ways takes over the regulatory function of the superego and becomes heir to the idealized parent of childhood. The reliance once vested in the parent now becomes attached to the self, and sacrifices of all kinds are made to sustain the sense of dignity and self-esteem.

Thus, inhibitory moral traditions do indeed have a function, one far more important and immediate than reproducing the genes. They serve as the vehicle of the transmission of culture from generation to generation. Within a generation, they serve to establish a sense of personal identity, a sense of integrity, and a sense of self-esteem.

When we consider the crisis of the professions in light of their cultural background, it becomes evident why the idea of a profession defined by a service ideal loses its credibility. Idealism in general has lost its credibility. Thus it becomes hard to imagine a profession in anything other than commercial terms because commerce has become the medium of social exchange. Put bluntly, the professions are being redefined as trades because the cultural structures that would support professional life are eroding. Since trust cannot be assumed, tighter regulation is deemed necessary, but in the process, the conditions for professional activity are undermined. Medicine is transformed from a human activity based on trust to a technical enterprise.

H. Tristram Engelhardt has suggested, not without regret, that the situation facing the modern physician is much like that facing the postman. The postman merely delivers what is called for, without judgment of value. The physician in a pluralistic society is merely a provider. The consumer shops for what is desired and in fact claims it as a personal right.[14].

In a culture of narcissism—that is to say, in a culture that does not provide the individual with a mirror of reality other than the expectation of grandiose wish-fulfillment without limitation—we see many of these wishes brought to the medical boutique. The expectations for medicine are so great that even mortality itself may be looked on as a failure of human achievement. We seem to expect perfect children, perfect health, and triumph over illness and death. Heinz Kohut in writing about the transformations of narcissism speaks of humor, empathy, wit, creativity, wisdom, and recognition of the finiteness of life.[15] His suggestion of the necessity of recognizing finitude is particularly timely for modern medicine in light of the sometimes grandiose expectations often placed on modern medicine.

Ethics can mediate conflicts that arise in this clash of expectations and can inform policy and daily practice. But it cannot do so in a cultural vacuum. It can provide a rational consideration of possible alternatives but it cannot stop at that. Ultimately ethics must be self-reflective. It must involve the self, the first person in the culture. Ethical reflection cannot substitute for the responsible actions of a moral agent. The final chapter looks at the meaning of responsible action for the physician.

CHAPTER 10

THE MEANING OF MEDICAL RESPONSIBILITY

S IR WILLIAM OSLER saw his profession as a balance between the art and science of medicine. He was worried even in his time that the balance was tipping toward science and that the legitimacy of the art of medicine was being undermined. Why should this have concerned him? Should this be a concern of ours?

I would like to go beyond the obvious answer to this question. We should be concerned not only because scientific medicine has created numerous ethical dilemmas arising from new technologies. An even more serious concern should be with the psychology of science, how it alters our thinking about our place in the world and particularly how it alters our thinking about professional activity. The question is not whether medicine should be scientific, but how it should be scientific. It should not be scientific in a way that undermines the humanistic aspects of medicine or transforms professionals into technicians.

If medicine is conceived as a scientific enterprise and if science is conceived as an impersonal understanding of nature, then medicine as a profession is transformed from the human service of the Oslerian ideal, science in the service of human need and defined by human goals, to an impersonal mechanism, human needs (and wants) being subsumed by biological norms understood in a statistical sense.

I realize that the point is controversial. Some would argue that biological norms must dictate the medical enterprise. Others would say that human beings have a right to self-determination, and therefore what they say must dictate what is done. Both positions are incomplete and miss the point. We must reclaim science as a human activity and must rethink our understanding of the professions in light of what we understand science or knowledge to be. This is obviously important for the medical profession, so closely identified with medical science, but it is no less important for any other profession in which expertise can be misunderstood as impersonal and value-neutral.

Let me illustrate the point succinctly before moving to a more detailed review of medical responsibility. Walker Percy, a physician-novelist who uses his medical background to diagnose the ills of our time, suggests the experience of the premedical student in dissecting the dogfish shark as a model of training the scientific mind. In dissecting the dogfish shark in the laboratory, one learns to look for features a particular dogfish has in common with all other dogfish. One learns not to attend to any features that might make a particular dogfish unique.[1]

Percy's example neatly encapsulates the problem of scientific education for the modern physician. The student physician has no concern for the uniqueness of the embalmed dogfish, but the living patient coming to the physician for help expects the physician to manifest that concern for personal uniqueness. This is an important part of the Oslerian ideal, the art of medicine, and there is no reason why scientific sophistication should preclude this human concern. We know, however, that patients often feel that they are but one in a series, and we know that in the press of time, physicians often resort to habits of thought learned while dissecting the dogfish.

Polanyi also speaks to this problem and also in medical metaphor. In his article, "Scientific Outlook: Its Sickness and Cure," he details the amorality of scientific detachment. He notes that:

> In the days when an idea could be silenced by showing that it was contrary to religion, theology was the greatest single source of fallacies. Today when any human thought can be discredited by branding it as unscientific, the power exercised previously by theology has passed over to science; hence, science has become in its turn the greatest single source of error.[2]

Polanyi had particular reasons for his concern about scientific dogmatism. He witnessed the dissolution of intellectual freedom in his native Hungary in the name of "scientific socialism," the morality of Marxist policy disguised as scientific theory.[3, 4, 5]

In order to help us appreciate the seductive familiarity of value-neutral accounts of moral situations in biology, sociology, and psychology, Polanyi offers numerous examples such as the following:

> Sociologists join forces here with psychiatrists in disguising their condemnation of social wrongs as the diagnosis of a mental disease. Thus, . . . when Hitler's rise fatally challenged our courage and intelligence, a whole literature of analytic treaties poured forth, propounding that wars were the result of pathological aggressiveness, caused mainly by training infants too soon to cleanliness.[6]

Obviously war is more than "tearing up 'scraps of paper', 'violating' an 'innocent little country', defending the 'mother' country, and more than fantasies of defense against the sinister (mostly sexual) designs of the fantasied 'bad' father."[7] Whether such accounts now seem insightful or foolish, they demonstrate the difficulty posed when moral judgment is obscured behind scientific observation. Psychoanalytic insight cuts very differently in the supportive environment of the professional's consulting room than it does as an account of external reality. Polanyi notes that he cites this literature not to make fun of its authors. "It should demonstrate on the contrary, that even the most distinguished minds can produce nothing truly relevant to human affairs if they restrict themselves by the kind of detachment which is currently supposed to be the mark of scientific integrity."[8]

Polanyi's antidote to this detachment is "participation." He suggests that we cannot study human society as though we were not part of it, but rather must participate in the human problems with which we are concerned. Certainly the physician is poised between the possibilities of detachment and participation in the life of those he or she serves. And the physician's effectiveness may well depend on how the professional role is understood either in terms of participation or detachment. As a scientist the physician may act in a detached manner, but only at the risk of not adequately responding to the person who has come for help. The professional must participate in the life of those served.

To the critic of modern medicine, it is not clear to what extent the activities of the profession are inspired by the Hippocratic tradition of patient benefit on the one hand or the ideal of scientific detachment inspired by biological norms. It is not clear whether the profession is defined by its ethics or its expertise. However much a particular physician may have been inspired by the Hippocratic tradition or the Oslerian ideal, a casual look at the overall landscape would suggest that a particular patient might well get caught up in the momentum of the medical mechanism with no real assurance that his or her own wishes would be heard, much less respected and acted upon.

Given this fear, it only makes sense to suggest that autonomy should be the overriding principle of medical ethics based on the right of self-determination of the rational individual. Given this fear, it only makes sense to view medical ethics in terms of informed consent. Medical paternalism seems antithetical to the desired autonomy, even though this paternalism is really more a feature of the Enlightenment ambition to control nature through science than it is the long-standing ideal of Hippocratic medicine.

A decade ago and throughout the history of medicine, physicians expected and were expected to be "paternalistic," to take responsibility for patients, to take care of them, even—and here is the problem—to decide on their behalf.[9] This nurturing aspect of medicine might equally well be called "maternalistic," even though most physicians have been male. Nonetheless the past decade has witnessed a dramatic rethinking about the attitude of paternalism, so that today paternalism has become a dirty word. Physicians, who once would have been concerned about being inadequately paternalistic and felt guilty about not doing enough for their patients, now are reluctant to assume this role for fear of being resented for their efforts. This development is not to be deplored insofar as it serves to provide greater equality in the health-care partnership. But just as excesses of paternalism must be kept in check, so also any attempt to make adversaries of physician and patient must be carefully scrutinized.

An example from a medical student paper will help focus the concerns young physicians are facing:

A 12-month-old baby was brought into the pediatric surgery room by his mother with a two-day history of fever, crying, and decreased appetite. Over the last several hours he had become increasingly irritable to the point that he could not be comforted by being held. He also resisted any efforts to move his head. On closer examination he was found to have an ear infection that had apparently developed into meningitis. Effective treatment required hospitalization and intravenous antibiotics. If accomplished rapidly, one is virtually always assured of a quick return to health without any aftereffects. In this case the mother was 15 years old, below the age of giving consent for her child although she desired treatment. Attempts to find the baby's grandmother were unsuccessful at first until neighbors finally located her at a tavern. Although she was not drunk, she was outraged that no one had informed her that "her baby" was being taken to the hospital and refused to give her permission for any intervention. After much persuasion, we finally succeeded in obtaining her consent. But in its absence, we were certainly prepared to admit the child, even if it meant securing the assistance of the hospital police to restrain the grandmother.[10]

The legal implications of conflicting rights and responsibilities complicate this case. Who really has and should have the right to consent or refuse to consent in this situation? The inevitable "paternalism" concerning the welfare of an infant is evident here. This student goes on to speculate how things might have been different if the patient were a different age:

I have often wondered what I would do in a similar situation involving a 24-year-old with probable meningitis who refused admission for himself because he wanted to die. Considering the probable results of no treatment, I'm sure that I would be prepared to take the same action. In the case of a 65-year-old with widely disseminated cancer and a similar infection, I might be more inclined to honor his refusal of treatment.

These situations pose some very important dilemmas for the physician, for the ethicist, for the law, and for society in general. Our idealized understanding of the working of informed consent presumes a rational (adult) mind, or in the case of an incompetent patient, a rational guardian. The grandmother, whose legal right it was to consent, was not acting rationally; she was offended because of an irrational claim she felt she had on her grandchild as "her baby." Yet if we know this family as people, we might find some legitimacy in the grandmother's claim as the one who in fact was parenting the baby. The medical student says he would be inclined to take the same action with a 24-year-old who wanted to die, presumably because the wish to die (in someone so young and otherwise healthy) could not be fully rational. The physician or student physician cannot be faulted for his concern for the patient, but might be faulted for attempting to force treatment on a supposedly rational adult.

The issue of patient autonomy becomes crucial for understanding how to practice medicine and how to reflect ethically on that practice. Patient autonomy and patients' rights are hot affective issues in contemporary medical ethical debate, and rightly so, for they identify concerns in our culture that go beyond the scope of medical practice.

Autonomy and paternalism are viewed as antithetical, mutually exclusive attitudes in medical practice and medical ethics. The paternalistic physician is seen as limiting patient autonomy; the autonomous patient is seen as not needing to be dependent on the physician. What is missing from this analysis is the dimension of time. The static formulations of physician as paternalistic or of patient as autonomous are characterizations that may approximate a given person at a particular instant, but say nothing about their relationship over time, its possibilities for change as the physician confronts the patient about undue dependency and unwillingness to get well, as the patient confronts the physician about undue withholding of information, and as they get to know each other and engage in dialogue, assessing and reassessing each other's needs and resources. It is this dynamic mutuality that may be said to characterize medical practice in the ideal sense of a partnership between physician and patient.

The complicating factor in this equilibrium is the issue of dependency. The patient may wish for dependency and at the same time fear it (and so may the physician). The wish/fear and the psychological defense against it/them may be so close as to be almost indistinguishable. It therefore makes sense to keep autonomy in mind as an ideal, not as an imperative to be administratively regulated. The physician does not refuse the patient's dependency wishes, but neither are those dependency wishes unduly gratified. Rather, they are temporarily accepted as part of the patient's sick role with the autonomy of the patient being the goal of the therapeutic approach.

The choice of the terms "autonomy" and "paternalism" and their opposition are somewhat unfortunate. Autonomy has too much the connotations of isolation and defensive, even defiant, refusal to affiliate with others. Paternalism has not only the masculine connotation, but the pejorative connotation of authoritarian control of another. It might be better to coin the neologism "parentalism" for the more caring and nurturing aspects of the doctor's concern for the patient. Just as responsible parents do not forever keep their children dependent but rather help them move toward independence, self-reliance, and autonomy, so the responsible physician accepts that at a time of illness the patient must inevitably be temporarily dependent on the physician as a person and on the skills the physician possesses. This neither implies that the physician is an omniscient/omnipotent god, nor does it imply that the physician must or should accede to the patient's every wish and demand.

Autonomy is generally seen as desirable, whereas dependency is seen as undesirable, at least in adults. This prejudice obviously creates problems in thinking about the dynamics of the doctor-patient relationship. The Japanese psychiatrist Takeo Doi has offered an analysis of dependency that is not only informative of Japanese character but of the experience of dependency, which receives little attention in Western thought.[11] The Japanese word *amae* describes the condition of passive love, for which European languages do not have an equivalent. *Amae* is the yearning to be taken care of. It is the experience of the infant at the breast. It may be the experience of the patient in time of suffering or illness.

I can best illustrate *amae* by describing my own experience of it in Japan. After meeting with Dr. Doi at Japan's National Institute of Mental Health, where he serves as its director, I was scheduled to give a lecture at one of the Tokyo universities. There was a conflict in scheduling, however, which would have prevented my accompanying my family on a sightseeing tour of the Japanese countryside. No problem, it was explained. I could give my lecture in Tokyo, then take the bullet train to catch up with my family at the first night's hotel.

After my lecture, I needed instructions to get to Tokyo station. A professor and a student accompanied me on the bus to the cross-city train and then on the train to Tokyo Station, then bought my ticket and accompanied me to the platform and onto the train. Not until they found a seat for me did they take their leave. What extraordinary courtesy to show a guest.

It was not until a couple of years later that I fully appreciated the cultural significance of this event. At the University of Oxford, I was introduced to a Japanese psychiatrist, Dr. Junichi Suzuki, an associate of Dr. Doi. After hearing about my experience, he asked simply, "Did you enjoy the regression?"

Schooled as I was in Western expectations of independence, autonomy, and Emersonian self-reliance, it had not occurred to me to "enjoy the regression." I realized that I had missed an opportunity to *amaeru*; that is, to behave self-indulgently. I did recall, however, a feeling of helpless dependence on my translator that could best be described as *amae*, though at the time "gratitude" was as close as I could come to describing the feeling.

Another example illustrates the importance of reorganizing dependence in caring for patients as persons, not just things. In distinguishing disease from illness, we found there were people who experienced illness for whom no disease could be identified. These people, often labeled pejoratively as "hysterics," seek dependency gratification and find that as patients they are able to appeal to the nurturing inclinations of family and physicians in ways that they (unconsciously) feel would not be possible for them if they were not "sick." Another group of patients is equally confounding for physicians, the group for whom disease is discovered but illness is not experienced, and who deny any need for help. The following case is representative:

A 42-year-old business executive is diagnosed as having hypertension at a routine physical examination. The executive is a vigorous and successful person for whom everything has gone well, he feels, because of his diligence and hard work. He was a successful student and athlete at an Ivy League college and rose to a major position in his company in a short period of time. He values self-reliance and industry. Though his work is stressful, he feels it causes him no undue problems and has been handling the responsibilities of his promotion without apparent difficulty.

The physician discusses with him the need to "slow down" and to change his lifestyle, and prescribes for him an antihypertensive medication, which he must take twice a day. They agree to a follow-up appointment six weeks later.

The executive does not keep the appointment, but four months later, he returns with increasingly severe headaches. The hypertension has become worse as manifested by both a higher blood pressure and perceptible symptoms.

This situation is common and perplexing to physicians and epidemiologists and there is a vast literature about the "noncompliant patient," which shows that there is no single personality type that can be identified as a noncompliant patient.[12] The 42-year-old executive is in many ways the opposite of the hysteric seeking dependency gratification through illness. He denies whatever dependency needs he has, including the very real need for help in "managing" or treating his life-threatening disease/illness. The fact that noncompliance is so widespread suggests that it is not a manifestation of a particular psychopathology but something universal in human experience. Again the presumption of human rationality is called into question, because if it were simply a rational matter, then the epidemiological arguments of the decreased longevity which accompanies hypertension and the relatively straightforward pharmacological means of treating it should at least make an impact on sophisticated patients like the executive and should be within the intellectual grasp of most people.

Obviously this is not simply a matter of rationality. The treatment of hypertension is a physiologically straightforward matter, but the treatment of a person with hypertension is much more complex. The decision of the patient to comply or not to comply with the physician's recommendations is not a decision that is made at any given instant, but a decision that is made time and again as the patient remembers or forgets to take the medicine. It is a temporally enduring series of decisions that involves not only epidemiological data and concerns about health and longevity, possibility of symptoms, and ultimately death, but also perception of oneself, a perception that may be altered by the physician's act of disclosing a diagnosis: "You are no longer a healthy person."

Thus the diagnosis of disease, even if not perceived as an illness, may involve a sense of loss for the patient, the loss of his or her identity as a healthy person. Following such a diagnosis, the patient may have to grieve the loss of the former self, following stages similar to those someone might pass through after the death of a spouse: denial, anger, and possibly depression, before coming to accept the loss.[13]

We can see that the 42-year-old executive with hypertension may be grieving the loss of his identity as a healthy, self-reliant, young man. The first stage of that grief is denial, probably at an irrational and unconscious level, reinforced by the fact that initially he experiences no symptoms. Were the physician sufficiently attuned to the biological-anthropological medical model, he might schedule an early return visit, anticipate the denial, and be prepared to help the patient voice his anger and frustration. Too often physicians (and nurses) discourage expressions of anger, which may be unfairly, or at least unreasonably, directed at them and their efforts to be helpful. Too often patients are reluctant to express anger, particularly towards someone on whom they may be dependent, for fear of being rejected. It is then that depression may become manifest, if the nature of the human experience of loss has not been discussed and clarified. Only then is it possible for the patient to accept the unpleasant reality and take whatever steps with the physician-partner that may be necessary to control the disease.

I offer this example to demonstrate the richness and complexity of events that may develop in the doctor-patient relationship over time. Even so straightforward a problem as hypertension, which can be conceived as a physiological problem, cannot rest on a treatment approach determined a priori, because both the disease and the patient who suffers with it are uniquely unpredictable. The physician must participate in the history of the patient and share it with the patient, hopefully changing it for the better over time. Any suggestion of a contractual model for the doctor-patient relationship based on patient autonomy, however desirable it is as a partial ideal, is ultimately misleading and limiting.[14] Any attempt to specify the particulars of a contract in advance, however much we are so tempted by our characteristic reliance on the Cartesian demand for explicitness, must inevitably fail because it ignores the richer, more complex, and more encompassing tacit dimension, on which explicitness ultimately depends.

Ethics may be conceived teleologically in terms of the articulation of certain principles that should underlie actions, and the effort must be made to articulate such principles. Ethics may also be conceived deontologically in terms of adherence to laws and rules, and certainly laws cannot be flouted if any stability in civilization is to be maintained. But both the principles and rules arise from a cultural situation, and this must also be understood, acknowledged, and accounted for in any attempt at right conduct.

H. Richard Niebuhr formulates this alternative approach to ethics under the concept of responsibility, which he points out includes the element of *response*, a response to the actions upon an individual in the cultural situation over time, so that ultimately responsibility involves a dialogue with others in a relationship that changes and develops over time. In summary of his argument he notes that

purposiveness seeks to answer the question: "What is my goal, ideal, or telos?" Deontology tries to answer the moral query by asking, first of all: "What is the law and what is the first law of my life?" Responsibility, however, proceeds in every moment of decision and choice to inquire: "What is going on?" If we use value terms then the differences among the three approaches may be indicated by the terms, the *good*, the *right*, and the *fitting*; for teleology is concerned always with the highest good to which it subordinates the right; consistent deontology is concerned with the right, no matter what may happen to our goods; but for the ethics of responsibility the fitting action, the one that fits into a total interaction as response and as anticipation of further response, is alone conducive to the good and alone is right.[15]

Niebuhr notes, as I have already suggested, that the question of responsibility is implied in the "primordial action of parental guidance: 'What is the fitting thing? What is going on in the life of the child?'"[16] Similarly the physician must ask at each stage of treatment, "What is going on in the life of the patient? How is this person experiencing his illness and what is his response to my prescriptions?"

Neither the physiological-technological approach to medicine nor the standard account of ethics fully accredits this personal, responsible, and ultimately moral approach to knowing and doing. This approach involves the cultural affairs of human beings, including the practice of medicine and the ethical reflection on that practice, as well as the various civic institutions of a culture—science, religion, morality, art, politics, marriage, family, or caring for children—any of the affairs of life that bring people into contact and interaction with one another.

Medicine needs the humanities just as it needs the sciences, not only to provide solutions to ethical dilemmas but also because the humanities teach one to deal with ambiguity, to make personal judgments, and to accept the responsibility for those judgments.

Descartes suggested that it might be possible to avoid all ambiguity that such human interaction entails, avoid affective unpleasantness, and avoid all dependence on others. It was a false promise, but a wish that mankind was so eager to accept that it was willing to sacrifice its sense of historical consciousness and its sense of the self as a moral agent capable of acting in history. The Cartesian outlook, a philosophical abbreviation for all those traditions sharing similar ideals, has never been unopposed. From the laments of Descartes's contemporary Blaise Pascal to modern phenomenology, psychoanalysis, epistemological revisionists such as Polanyi and moral philosophers such as John Macmurray, and theologians such as H. Richard Niebuhr and Stanley Hauerwas, a vigorous opposition movement has insisted that humans continue to occupy a special place in the universe, if not as an extension of God or pinnacle of creation, then certainly as a locus of self-awareness and source of responsible action.

The analysis of medical ethics in terms of the relationship between the doctor and the patient suggests analogous considerations for other civic institutions and for other relationships between people, including sexual relationships, marriage, family, and childrearing or parenting. Focus on the rights of individuals without adequate attention to the personal responsibility to others engenders an adversarial stance and reveals the narcissistic expectations of self-gratification. This departure from a fiduciary partnership substitutes an appeal to "ethics" as the basis for a demand made on another. We have come to recognize that not every appeal to ethics is necessarily ethical, and morality can be inverted for interests that also claim to be moral.

Thus ethics as a discipline shares with medicine as a profession and any citizen of our culture striving to be moral, allegiances to standards that no human being can possibly live up to. This does not mean that anything goes, or that values are just relative. It may be concluded, however, that one should practice ethics, just as one should practice medicine, not with a sense of self-satisfaction, but with respect for the limitations inherent in the human condition and with humility.

Medicine as a profession is identified with ideals of human service that can be neither completely specified nor ultimately fulfilled. To a society expecting complete explicitness in all relationships, any idealistic notion of a profession seems incredible. Yet there remain expectations of personal attention and service. The physician strives to be trustworthy, recognizing the various needs, wishes, and expectations that the patient may bring to the encounter. Medicine is inherently ambiguous, because it is a human enterprise.

Medicine may be defined by the ambiguous and manifestly imperfect ideal of human service or by an apparently more precise science or technology, but the apparent precision of science is delusive. Polanyi reminds us that life cannot be explained according to the laws of physics and chemistry, in contradiction to the tenets of most physiology texts. "When I say that life transcends physics and chemistry, I mean that biology cannot explain life in our age by the current working of physical and chemical laws."[17] Even though the human body may be understood as a machine, the workings of a machine cannot be explained by physics and chemistry. The meaning and purpose of a grandfather clock, for example, cannot be understood by an explanation of its components. Furthermore, the laws of physics and chemistry would still apply even if the machine were smashed to bits. It is human judgment that determines meaning.

This is an important clarification for modern medicine and medical ethics. Much of medicine's success has come from its ability to look at ever lower levels of biological organization, the organism, the cell, the molecule. But understanding the parts does not justify the purposes or provide meaning. Psychiatry as a profession is also caught up in this misunderstanding. For psychiatry as for the rest of medicine to be truly scientific and truly biological, it must give an account of its understanding of the meaning and purpose of life, not just the workings of molecules. For psychiatry as for the rest of medicine to be professional it must speak to human needs and human ideals as well as specific techniques, be those techniques psychological or biological. The medical model is necessarily biological-anthropological in the broadest sense of understanding human meaning and purposes. It is toward the end of remembering this important aspect of professional life that this book is directed.

Endnotes

INTRODUCTION

1. Pincoffs, Edmund: Quandary ethics. *Mind* 75:552–571, October 1971.
2. Hauerwas, Stanley: *Community and Character*. Notre Dame: University of Notre Dame Press, 1981.
3. Douglas Adams and Phil Mullins argue along similar lines in "Conscience, tacit knowledge, and the art of judgment: implications of Polanyi's thought for moral reflection." *Soundings* 66(1):34–45, 1983.
4. See Dyer, Allen R.: The dreams of Descartes: notes on the origins of scientific thinking. *Annual of Psychoanalysis* 14:163–175, 1986.
5. Polanyi, Michael: *Personal Knowledge: Towards a Post-Critical Philosophy*. New York: Harper and Row, 1964, p. xi.
6. Polanyi, p. xiii.
7. Larry R. Churchill argues along similar lines in his paper, "Bioethical reductionism and our sense of the human," *Man and Medicine* 5(4):229–242, 1980. See also Smith, Harmon L., and Larry R. Churchill: *Professional Ethics and Primary Care Medicine*. Durham, NC: Duke University Press, 1986.
8. Anecdote supplied by Willard Gaylin, personal communication.
9. Veatch, Robert: The generalization of expertise. *The Hastings Center Studies* 1:29–40, 1973.
10. See also Leon Kass's essays, "Is there a medical ethic?: the Hippocratic Oath and the sources of ethical medicine," in *Toward a More Natural Science: Biology and Human Affairs*. New York: The Free Press, 1985.
11. Guttentag, Otto E.: On defining medicine. *The Christian Scholar* 46:200–211, 1963.
12. Engel, George: The need for a new medical model: a challenge for biomedicine. *Science* 196:129–136, 1977.

CHAPTER 1

1. Campbell, Dennis: *Doctors, Lawyers, Ministers*. Nashville: Abingdon, 1982, pp. 17–26.
2. La Vopa, Anthony J.: Humanism and professional education: historical background, in *The Humanities and the Profession of Medicine*. Edited by Allen R. Dyer. Research Triangle Park, NC: National Humanities Center, 1982, pp 1–23.
3. Post, Seymour G.: Parisian masters as a corporation, 1200–1246. *Spectrum* 9:421–445, 1934.
4. Thrupp, S. L.: *The Guilds, Cambridge Economic History of Europe*. Cambridge: Cambridge University Press, 1963.
5. Moline, Jon: On professionals and professions, in *The Humanities and the*

Profession of Medicine Research. Edited by Allen R. Dyer. Research Triangle Park, NC: National Humanities Center, 1982, pp. 45–65.
6. Reiser, Stanley J., Arthur J. Dyck, and William J. Curran (eds.): *Ethics in Medicine:Historical Perspectives and Contemporary Concerns.* Cambridge, MA: MIT Press, 1977, p. 1.
7. Michels, Robert: Professional ethics and social value. *International Review of Psychoanalysis* 3:377–384, 1976.
8. Friedson, E.: *Profession of Medicine: A Study of the Sociology of Applied Knowledge.* New York: Dodd, Mead, 1970.
9. Larson, M. S.: *The Rise of Professionalism: A Sociological Analysis.* Berkeley: University of California Press, 1977.
10. Haskell, T. L.: *The Emergence of Professional Social Science.* Urbana: University of Illinois Press, 1977.
11. Wilensky, H.: The professionalization of everyone? *The American Journal of Sociology* 70:137ff, 1964.
12. Weber, Max: *On the Methodology of the Social Sciences.* Translated and edited by E. A. Shils and H. A. Finch. Glencoe: The Free Press, 1949.
13. Berlant, Jeffrey: *Profession and Monopoly: A Study of Medicine in the United States and Great Britain.* Berkeley: University of California Press, 1975.
14. Greenhouse, J.: Justices uphold right of doctors to solicit trade. *The New York Times,* 24 March 1982, p. 10.
15. Lee, R. E.: Application of antitrust laws to the professions. *Journal of Legal Medicine* 1(2):143–153, 1979.
16. Havighurst, Clark: Antitrust enforcement in the medical services industry: what does it all mean? *Milbank Memorial Fund Quarterly/Health and Society* 58(1):89–124, 1980.
17. Pertschuk, Michael B.: FTC Conference, June 1–2, 1977. Quoted in Rosoff, A.J.: Antitrust laws and the health care industry: new warriors into an old battle. *Saint Louis University Law Journal* 23:478, 1979. Also quoted in Ballantine, H. Thomas, Jr.: Annual discourse—the crisis in ethics, anno domini 1979. *New England Journal of Medicine* 301:634, 1979.
18. Relman, Arthur S.: Professional directories—but not commercial advertising—as a public service. *New England Journal of Medicine* 29:476–478, 1978.
19. Christians, C. G., Q. J. Schultze, and N. H. Simms: Community, epistemology, and mass media ethics. *Journalism History* 5:38–41, 65–67, 1978.
20. Schultze, Q. J.: Professionalism in advertising: The origin of ethical codes. *Journal of Communication* 31:64–71, 1981.

CHAPTER 2

1. Carrick, Paul: *Medical Ethics in Antiquity.* Boston: D. Reidel, 1985, p. 158.
2. References to the oath are to the Edelstein translation (the Oath attributed to Hippocrates, pagan version, as translated by Ludwig Edelstein). Edelstein, Ludwig: The Hippocratic Oath. Text, translation, and interpretation. *Bulletin of the History of Medicine* (Supplement no. 1); 1943, p. 3. Also in Edelstein, L.: *Ancient Medicine.* Baltimore: Johns Hopkins University Press, 1967.
3. Konold, Donald: Codes of medical ethics, in *Encyclopedia of Medical Ethics,* vol. 1. New York: The Free Press, 1978, p. 163.

4. Mead, Margaret: Personal communication to Maurice Levine, 1961. Cited in Levine, *Psychiatry & Ethics*, New York: George Braziller, 1972, pp. 324–325.
5. Konold, in *Encyclopedia of Medical Ethics*, p. 163.
6. *Decorum* XVI, in Carrick, p. 183.
7. Altman, Lawrence K.: The doctor's world. *The New York Times*, 1 May 1979, p. CL. Quoted in Chapman, Carlton B.: *Physicians, Law and Ethics*. New York: New York University Press, 1984.
8. Chapman, Carlton B.: *Physicians, Law and Ethics*. New York: New York University Press, 1984, p. 179.
9. Leake, Chauncey: *Percival's Medical Ethics*. Baltimore: Williams & Wilkins, 1927, pp. 1–2.
10. Carrick, p. 175.
11. Veatch, Robert: *A Theory of Medical Ethics*. New York: Basic Books, 1981, pp. 15–26.
12. Carrick, p. 180.
13. Edelstein translation. See reference 2.
14. Levine, Maurice: *Psychiatric & Ethics*. New York: George Braziller, 1972, pp. 323–341.

CHAPTER 3

1. Freedman, Daniel X. Cited in Romano, J.: Reflections on informed consent. *Archives of General Psychiatry* 30:192–235, 1974. This distinction is originally attributable to the German sociologist F. Toennies, *Fundamental Concepts of Sociology*. Translated by Charles Loomis. New York: America Book Company, 1940.
2. Leake, Chauncey: *Percival's Medical Ethics*. Baltimore: Williams & Wilkins, 1927, pp. 1–2.
3. Clouser, K. Danner: What is medical ethics? *Annals of Internal Medicine* 80:657–660, 1974.
4. Moore, Charles B.: *This* is medical ethics? *The Hastings Center Report*, 4(5):1–3, 1974. The Hastings Center is the Institute of Society, Ethics and the Life Sciences in Hastings, New York.
5. Prior to World War II one could cite religious texts such as the Decalogue, the Oath of Hippocrates, and Thomas Percival's *Code of Medical Ethics* (1803), but basically medical ethics derived from tacitly understood religious and cultural traditions. While many of these traditions are still valid and valued, the list of guidelines with which a physician now must be familiar is extensive and includes the following: The "Principles of Medical Ethics" of the American Medical Association, Opinions and Reports of the Judicial Council (AMA); "The Nuremburg Code (1947)"; the Declaration of Helsinki, adopted in 1964 by the World Medical Association; "the Institutional Guide to DHEW Policy on Protection of Human Subjects" (NIH)72-102, published in 1971; and the American Hospital Association's 12-point Patient's Bill of Rights. The rate of increase in the number of federal and state statutes and the trend of recent judicial decisions really necessitate specialized legal consultation for a current appraisal of acceptable conduct in particular situations.

151

6. Reiser, Stanley J., Arthur J. Dyck, and William J. Curran, eds.: *Ethics in Medicine: Historical Perspectives and Contemporary Concerns.* Cambridge, MA: MIT Press, 1977, p. 1.
7. It is interesting to realize that although we think today of a profession as being defined by the knowledge of a learned science, originally a profession was the verbal profession of vows upon entering a religious order. I wish to stress this point because I do not believe things have really changed that much if one considers what knowledge is in the continuity of human ideas. In medieval times knowledge was the province of religious orders, but modern science had its origins in religious belief. Even in modern times there is an ingredient of personal commitment to the things known or believed, which is generally ignored in our contemporary accounts of science.
8. Frankena, William: *Ethics.* Englewood, Cliffs, NJ: Prentice-Hall, 1963.
9. Fletcher, Joseph: *Situation Ethics.* Philadelphia: Westminister Press, 1966; *Morals and Medicine.* Princeton: Princeton University Press, 1954.
10. The decision trees are reproduced with permission from Howard Brody's excellent programmed text, *Ethical Decisions in Medicine*, Boston: Little, Brown, 2nd edition 1981.
11. Kant, Immanuel: *Fundamental Principles of the Metaphysic of Morals.* Indianapolis: The Library of Liberal Arts, Bobbs-Merill, 1949, p. 38.
12. Kant, p. 46.
13. Hauerwas, Stanley: *Truthfulness and Tragedy.* Notre Dame: University of Notre Dame Press, 1977, p. 2. See also Pincoffs, Edmund: Quandary ethics. *Mind* 75:552–571, October 1971.
14. Frankena, William: Pritchard and the ethics of virtue. *The Monist* 54:17, 1970. Quoted in Hauerwas, *Truthfulness and Tragedy*, p. 40.
15. Hauerwas, p. 41.
16. Edel, Abraham: *Ethical Judgment: The Use of Science in Ethics.* New York: The Free Press, 1964, p. 15.
17. Scriven, Michael: *The Science of Ethics*, p. 39. Quoted in Campbell, Donald: Response to Dyer. *American Psychologist*, 33:770–772, 1978. See Appendix to Chapter 2 for the context of this debate.

CHAPTER 4

1. *Tarasoff v. Regents of University of Cal.*, 17 Cal. 3d 425 (1976).
2. See Winslade, William J., and Judith W. Ross: Privacy, confidentiality, and autonomy in psychotherapy. *Nebraska Law Review* 64(4):578–636, 1985.
3. Heyman, Gary M.: Mandated child abuse reporting and the confidentiality privilege, in *Psychotherapy and the Law.* Edited by Louis Everstine and Diana Sullivan Everstine. Orlando, FL: Grune and Stratton, 1986, pp. 145–155.
4. *Raleigh News and Observer*, 13 February 1986, p. 1C, and *Durham Morning Herald*, 12 February 1986, p. 1.
5. Heyman, in *Psychotherapy and the Law*, pp. 152–154.
6. Thompson, Ian E.: "The Nature of Confidentiality," *Journal of Medical Ethics*, 1979, 5, p.62.

CHAPTER 5

1. See Nader, Ralph, and Sidney Wolfe: Is the American health system bad for America's health? *Practical Psychology for Physicians*, December 1976, pp. 30–38. Illych, Ivan: *Medical Nemesis*. New York: Pantheon Books, 1976; and Szasz, Thomas: *The Myth of Mental Illness*. New York: Harper and Row, 1974.
2. Guttentag, Otto E.: The attending physician as central figure, in *Changing Values in Medicine*. Edited by Eric J. Cassell and Mark Siegler. Chicago: University Publications of America, 1979, pp. 107–126. Also see Care of the healthy and the sick from the attending physician's perspective: envisioned and actual, in *Organism Medicine and Metaphysics*. Edited by S. F. Spicker. Dordrecht, Holland: D. Reidel, 1978, pp. 41–56. Alternatively, to enlarge the scope of biology to encompass the study of life, we might distinguish the biological-technological medical model from the biological-anthropological medical model.
3. As an example of the materialistic problems associated in medical ethics, we may consider attempts to resolve ethical dilemmas in medicine by identifying life in mechanical or physiological terms. These problems often appear as attempts to "define" life or death. When may an artificial respirator be turned off, for example? At first glance it might appear that a new definition of death might make this decision easier, but the issues involved are not technical in nature but personal. For a detailed discussion of the ethical and legal issues involved in such a decision, my article "Natural Death in Medical Practice" provides more detail than is possible here. (See Dyer, Allen R., and William B. Bunn: Natural death in medical practice. *North Carolina Medical Journal* 41:147–151, 1980.

    Abortion is another particularly distressing example of a situation in which the conflicting values of our culture are camouflaged as concern about the definition and origin of life. The abortion debate involves many issues simultaneously, including the rights of a woman to self-determination of her body; the potential rights of a fetus to life; attitudes toward sex; reproduction and responsibility for offspring; knowledge of the consequences, physical and emotional, of sexual intercourse; birth control, family planning, and population limitation in an overcrowded world. The debate does not, however, involve the definition of life, which is an issue almost irrelevant to the passions that stir the debate. It is ironic that we are asked to consider this moral issue in terms that equate life with cellular metabolism, when the concern is how to assess the value of human life. No one would base an ethical argument on the "right to cellular metabolism" when by human life we understand so much more. Though space does not permit the examination these issues warrant, they need to be identified in the context of our understanding of what a person is and what medicine's responsibility to that person is.
4. Guttentag, Otto E.: On defining medicine. *The Christian Scholar* 46:200–211, 1963.
5. See Eisenberg, Leon: Disease and illness: distinctions between professional and popular ideas of Sickness. *Culture, Medicine and Psychiatry* 1:9–23, 1977.
6. Engelhardt, H. Tristram, Jr.: The disease of masturbation: values and the

concept of disease. *Bulletin of Historical Medicine* 48:234–248, 1974.

7. Engel, George: The need for a new medical model: a challenge for biomedicine. *Science* 196:129–136, 1977.

8. Szasz, Thomas: *The Myth of Mental Illness*. New York: Harper and Row, 1974, p. 267.

9. Freud, Sigmund: On the history of psychoanalytic movement (1914), in *The Complete Psychological Works of Sigmund Freud, Standard Edition*, vol. 14. Translated and Edited by James Strachey. London: The Hogarth Press and the Institute of Psycho-Analysis, 1957, pp. 13–14. Quoted in Szasz, *The Myth of Mental Illness*, pp. 21–22.

10. Szasz, p. 73.

11. Breuer, Joseph, and Sigmund Freud: *Studies on Hysteria* (1893–1895), pp. 143–144. Quoted in Szasz, *The Myth of Mental Illness*, p. 73.

12. There can be no question, however, that Freud equivocates on the relationship between the psychological and physical sciences. He strove to be scientific and succeeded, not because he offered physical explanations for mental phenomena, but because he offered an explanatory system based on his careful observations, which were "real" and "believable." His reliance on mechanical metaphors stated as fact continues to be a point of contention in Freudian criticism and interpretation. The working psychoanalyst is successful, just as the working physicist is successful, by ignoring the would-be explanations of a strictly quantitative positivist philosophy. A psychoanalyst comes by his understanding of the historical antecedents (or "determinants") of adult rationality as much through his own experience in personal psychoanalysis as through a study of the writings of others. A literary critic or philosopher, however, who tries to understand Freud strictly through his writings may be seriously misled about the meaning of such concepts as "overdetermination," for example, which was Freud's creative equivocation for saying that although there are many antecedent "causes" for the things people experience, these causes do not have a strict cause-and-effect relationship: There are too many determinants to permit quantification.

13. A system that does adequately account for these tensions is that of Paul Tillich in *Love, Power and Justice: Ontological Analyses and Ethical Applications* (New York: Oxford University Press, 1954) or his *Systematic Theology* (Chicago: University of Chicago Press, 1951–1963), in which he discusses "finite freedom." Finite freedom is fundamentally a recognition of our own mortality and of the limitations inherent in the human condition. The wish for absolute freedom, on the other hand, is a remnant of our infantile narcissism, the grandiose desire that our impulses not be bound by the limitations of necessity and the reality principle.

14. Bok, Sissela: *Lying: Moral Choice in Public and Private Life*. New York: Pantheon Books, 1978, p. 11.

15. Poteat, William: *Polanyian Meditations*. Durham, NC: Duke University Press, 1986.

CHAPTER 6

1. Redlich, Fritz, and Richard Mollica: Overview: ethical issues in contemporary psychiatry. *American Journal of Psychiatry* 133(2): 125–136, 1976.

1. Redlich, Fritz, and Richard Mollica: Overview: ethical issues in contemporary psychiatry. *American Journal of Psychiatry* 133(2): 125–136, 1976.
2. Riskin, L.: Informed consent: looking for the action. *University of Illinois Law Forum* 4:580–611, 1975.
3. Mills, M. J., L. C. Hsu, and P. A. Berger: Informed consent: psychotic patients and research. *Bulletin of the American Academy of Psychiatry and the Law* 8:119–132, 1980.
4. Zerubavel, E.: The bureaucratization of responsibility: the case of informed consent. *Bulletin of the American Academy of Psychiatry and the Law* 8:161–167, 1980.
5. Strong, Carson: Informed consent: theory and practice. *Journal of Medical Ethics* 5:196–199, 1979.
6. Lebacqz, Karen, and Robert J. Levine: Respect for persons and informed consent to participate in research. *Clinical Research* 25:101–107, 1977.
7. Gray, B. H.: Complexities of informed consent. *Annals of the American Academy of Political Science* 437:37–48, 1978.
8. Veatch, Robert: Three theories of informed consent: philosophical foundations and policy implications. The National Commission for the Protection of Human Subjects of Biomedical and Behavioral Research (The Belmont Report), 1976.
9. Erikson, Erik: *Identity and the Lifecycle.* Psychological Issues Monograph Series, vol. 1, no. 1. New York: International Universities Press, 1959.
10. Mahler, Margaret S., Fred Pine, and Anni Bergman: *The Psychological Birth of the Human Infant: Symbiosis and Individuation.* New York: Philosophical Library, 1944.
11. Beauchamp, Thomas, and James Childress: *Principles of Biomedical Ethics.* New York: Oxford University Press, 1979, pp. 67–68.
12. Appelbaum, P.S., and L.H. Roth: Clinical Issues in the Assessment of Competency. *American Journal of Psychiatry* v138:1462-1467 Nov 1981.
13. Stanley, B. H., and M. Stanley: Psychiatric patients in research: protecting their autonomy. *Comprehensive Psychiatry* 22:420–427, 1981.
14. Guttentag, Otto E.: Ethical problems in human experimentation, in *Ethical Issues in Medicine.* Edited by E. F. Torrey. Boston: Little, Brown, 1968, pp. 197–226.
15. Guttentag, Ethical problems in human experimentation, pp. 197–226.
16. Guttentag, Otto E.: The problem of experimentation on human beings: the physician's point of view. *Science* 117:205, 1953.
17. Dyer, Allen R.: Informed consent and the non-autonomous person. *IRB: A Review of Human Subjects Research* 4:1–4, 1982.
18. Appelbam and Roth *Ibid.*
19. Whitehead, T.: *Mental Illness and the Law.* New York: Basil Blackwell, 1983.
20. *All England Law Reports,* 1984, pp. 1018–1036.
21. *All England Law Reports,* 1984, p. 1031.
22. *All England Law Reports,* 1984, pp. 1030–1031.
23. *All England Law Reports,* 1984, p. 1036.
24. *All England Law Reports,* 1984, p. 1044.
25. Bai, Koichi: Patients' autonomy in Japan viewed in terms of consent. ACTA, Sixth World Congress on Medical Law. Gent, August 22–26, 1982, Deel 2, pp. 7–11.
26. Bai, pp. 7–11.

CHAPTER 7

1. Sider, Roger C., and Colleen Clements: Psychiatry's contribution to medical ethics education. *American Journal of Psychiatry* 139(4):498–501, 1982.
2. Freud, Sigmund: Freud's psychoanalytic procedure (1900), in *The Complete Psychological Works of Sigmund Freud, Standard Edition*, vol. 7. Translated and Edited by James Strachey. London: The Hogarth Press and the Institute of Psycho-Analysis, 1957, p. 254.
3. Fromm, Erich: *Man for Himself: An Inquiry into the Psychology of Ethics.* New York: Holt, Rinehart, and Winston, 1947, p. 42.
4. Girouard, M.: The public schools, in *The Return to Camelot: Chivalry and the English Gentleman*. New Haven and London: Yale University Press, 1981, p. 169.
5. Thomas Arnold, in *Encyclopaedia Britannica*, vol. 2, 1951, p. 425.
6. Freud, Sigmund: Interpretation of dreams (1900), in *Standard Edition*, vol. 4, pp. 1–338.
7. Freud, Sigmund: Three essays on the theory of sexuality (1905), in *Standard Edition*, vol. 7, pp. 238–239.
8. Freud, Sigmund: Character and anal erotism (1908), in *Standard Edition*, vol. 9, pp. 167–175.
9. Abraham, K.: Contributions to the theory of the anal character, in *Selected Papers of Karl Abraham*. London: Maresfield Reprints, 1927.
10. Freud, Sigmund: The disposition to obsessional neurosis (1913), in *Standard Edition*, vol. 12, pp. 317–325.
11. Reich, Wilhelm: *Character Analysis*. London: Vision Press, 1949, p. 318.
12. American Psychiatric Association: *Diagnostic and Statistical Manual of Mental Disorders, Third Edition*. Washington, DC: American Psychiatric Association, 1980.
13. Reich, *Character Analysis*, p. 318.
14. Auchincloss, E., and R. Michels: Psychoanalytic theory of character, in *Current Perspectives on Personality Disorders*. Edited by J. Frosch. Washington, DC: American Psychiatric Press, 1983.
15. Kaplan, A.: Freud and modern philosophy, in *Freud and the 20th Century*. Edited by B. Nelson. New York: Meridian Books, 1957, pp. 209–223.
16. Polanyi, Michael: *Personal Knowledge: Towards a Post-Critical Philosophy*. New York: Harper and Row, 1964.
17. *Principles of Medical Ethics with Annotations Applicable to Psychiatry.* Washington, DC: American Psychiatric Press, 1986.

CHAPTER 8

1. Dostoevsky, Fyodor: *The Brothers Karamazov*. Cited in Edel, Abraham: *Ethical Judgment: The Use of Science in Ethics*. New York: The Free Press, 1964.
2. This case is adapted from Howard Brody's book, *Ethical Decisions in Medicine* (Boston: Little, Brown, 1976).
3. Maugham, Somerset: *Points of View*. Quoted in Castelnuovo-Tedesco, Pietro: "The mind as a stage." Some comments on reminiscence and internal

objects. *International Journal of Psychoanalysis* 59:19, 1978.

4. Merleau-Ponty, Maurice: *Phenomenology of Perception*. London: Routledge and Kegan-Paul, 1962, p. 410ff.

5. Piaget, Jean: *La Representation du monde chez l'enfant*. Cited in Merleau-Ponty, *Phenomenology of Perception*, p. 355.

6. Piaget, *La Representation du monde chez l'enfant*, p. 21. Cited in Merleau-Ponty, Maurice: *Phenomenology of Perception*. For further discussion, see my article "R. D. Laing in Post-Critical Perspective," *British Journal of Psychiatry* 124:252–259, March 1974.

7. Macmurray, John: *The Self as Agent*. London: Faber, 1957, p. 21.

8. Macmurray, p. 23.

9. Ryle, Gilbert: *The Concept of Mind*. London: Hutchison, 1949.

10. Etymologically "emotion" is derived from the Old French, *esmovoir*, to excite, and from the Latin, *emovere*, to move out, stir up, excite.

11. Freud, Sigmund: On narcissism: an introduction (1914–1916), in *The Complete Psychological Works of Sigmund Freud, Standard Edition*, vol. 14. Translated and Edited by James Strachey. London: The Hogarth Press and the Institute of Psycho-Analysis, 1957, pp. 203–204. One of the best and most succinct discussions of narcissism appears in my wife's Ph.D. dissertation: Susan K. Dyer, *Plinlimmon's Theme: The Aspirations and Limitations of Man in the Novels of Herman Melville* (Durham, NC: Duke University, 1977) (available from University Microfilms, Ann Arbor, Michigan). Also the writings of Heinz Kohut, particularly *The Analysis of the Self* (New York: International Universities Press, 1971), and Otto Kernberg, particularly *Borderline Conditions and Pathological Narcissism* (New York: Jason Aronson, 1971), have stimulated much interest and rethinking of the psychoanalytic theories of narcissism.

12. Freud, The ego and the id (1923–1925), in *Standard Edition*, vol. 14, pp. 3–66.

13. Freud, Totem and taboo (1913–1914), in *Standard Edition*, vol. 13, pp. 1–165.

14. Freud, Group psychology and the analysis of the ego (1921), in *Standard Edition*, vol. 18, p. 110.

15. Hartmann, H., and R. Lowenstein: Notes on the superego. *Psychoanalytic Study of the Child* 17:1, 1962.

16. Freud, Neurosis and psychosis (1924), in *Standard Edition*, vol. 19, pp. 92–93.

17. Freud, Civilization and its discontents (1930), in *Standard Edition*, vol. 21, pp. 64–145.

18. Gilligan, James: Beyond morality: psychoanalytic reflections on shame, guilt and love, in *Moral Development and Behavior: Theory, Research, and Social Issues*. Edited by Thomas Likona. New York: Holt, Rinehart and Winston, 1976, pp. 144–158. See also Piers G. and M. Singer: *Shame and Guilt*. Springfield, IL: Charles C. Thomas, 1953.

19. Benedict, R.: *Patterns of Culture*. New York: New American Library, 1958, p. 198. Cited in Gilligan, in *Moral Development and Behavior*, p. 146.

20. Kaplan J., and T. Plaut: *Personality in a Communal Society*. Lawrence: University of Kansas, 1956, p. 12. Cited in Gilligan, in *Moral Development and Behavior*.

21. For an excellent analysis of the concept of agency, see Rogers, William R.:

157

Helplessness and agency in the healing process. in *Nourishing the Humanistic in Medicine: Interactions with the Social Sciences*. Edited by William R. Rogers and David Bernard. Pittsburgh: University of Pittsburgh Press, 1979, pp. 25–52.

22. Polanyi, Michael: *Personal Knowledge: Towards a Post-Critical Philosophy*. New York, Harper and Row, 1964, pp. 230–235.
23. Polanyi, p. 12.
24. Polanyi, p. 230.

CHAPTER 9

1. Lasch, Christopher: *The Culture of Narcissism: American Life in an Age of Diminishing Expectations*. New York: Norton, 1978.
2. Comte, Auguste: *System of Positive Polity*, 4 vols. London: Longmans, Green and Company, 1875–1877.
3. For an excellent review of this epoch of American history see Budd, Louis: Altruism arrives in america. *American Quarterly* 8:40–52, Spring 1956.
4. Ghiselin, M. T.: *The Economy of Nature and the Evolution of Sex*. Berkeley: University of California Press, 1974. (This is the very sentiment to which Polanyi calls attention in his discussion of the moral inversion. It is the ideals that have been called altruistic that are inverted.)
5. Wilson, E. O.: *Sociobiology: The New Synthesis*. Cambridge: Belknap/Harvard University Press, 1975; Barsch, David P.: *Sociobiology and Behavior*, New York: Elsevier, 1977; Dawkins, Gerald: *The Selfish Gene*, New York, Oxford, 1976.
6. Polanyi, Michael: *Personal Knowledge: Towards a Post-Critical Philosophy*. New York: Harper and Row, 1964, p. 16.
7. Campbell, Donald: On the conflicts between biological and social evolution and between psychology and moral tradition. *American Psychologist* 30:1103–1126, 1975.
8. Campbell, p. 1103.
9. Campbell, p. 1104.
10. Menninger, Karl: *Whatever Became of Sin?* New York: Hawthorn, 1973.
11. Campbell, p. 1116.
12. See Hamilton, Edith: *Mythology*. Boston: Little, Brown, 1942.
13. See Lasch, *The Culture of Narcissism*.
14. Engelhardt, H. Tristram Jr.: The disease of masturbation: values and the concept of disease. *Bulletin of Historical Medicine* 48:234–248, 1974.
15. Kohut, Heinz: *The Analysis of the Self*. New York: International Universities Press, 1971.

CHAPTER 10

1. Percy, Walker: The diagnostic novel. *Harper's Magazine*, June 1986, pp. 39–45.
2. Polanyi, Michael: Scientific outlook: its sickness and cure. *Science* 125:480–484, 1957.

3. Polanyi, Scientific outlook, pp. 480–484.
4. Polanyi, Michael: The message of the Hungarian revolution. *Christianity and Crisis*, 31 October 1966, pp. 240–243.
5. Polanyi, Michael: The message of the Hungarian revolution. *The American Scholar* 35:661–676, Autumn 1966.
6. Polanyi, Scientific outlook, p. 482.
7. Glover, E.: *War, Sadism and Pacifism*. London: George Allen and Unwin, Ltd., 1933. Cited in Polanyi, Scientific outlook, p. 484.
8. Polanyi, Scientific outlook, p. 482.
9. There is an important difference between the legal and medical concepts of trust. In law, a fiduciary stands for the client and decides in the client's best interests. In medicine, the physician is expected to decide in partnership with the patient.
10. Crimm, Allan, and Raymond Greenberg: Reflections on the doctor-patient relationship: paternalism and autonomy, in *Ethical Dimensions of Clinical Medicine*. Edited by Allen R. Dyer and Dennis A. Robbins. Springfield, IL: Charles Thomas Publishers, 1981, pp. 104–110.
11. Doi, Takeo: *The Anatomy of Dependence*. Tokyo: Kodanska International, 1981.
12. Houpt, J., C. Orleans, L. George, and H. K. H. Brodie: *The Importance of Mental Health Services for General Health Care*. Cambridge, MA: Ballinger Press, 1979, p. 203.
13. George Engel is also helpful on this point in his discussion of when grief is an illness. See "The need for a new medical model: A challenge for biomedicine," *Science* 196:129–131, 1977.
14. See Veatch, Robert: The medical model: its nature and problems, *The Hastings Center Studies* 3:59–76, 1973.
15. Niebuhr, H. Richard: *The Responsible Self: An Essay in Christian Moral Philosophy*. New York: Harper and Row, 1963, pp. 60–61.
16. Niebuhr, p. 60.
17. Polanyi, Michael: Life transcending physics and chemistry. *Chemical and Engineering News* 45:55–66, 1967.

BIBLIOGRAPHY

Abraham, Karl: Contributions to the theory of anal character, in *Selected Papers of Karl Abraham*. 1921. Reprint. London: Maresfield Reprints, 1927.

Adams, Douglas, and Phil Mullins: Conscience, tacit knowledge, and the art of judgment: implications of Polanyi's thought for moral reflection. *Soundings* 66(1):34–45, 1983.

All England Law Reports, 1984.

Altman, Lawrence K.: The doctor's world. *The New York Times*, 1 May 1979, p. CL.

American Psychiatric Association: *Diagnostic and Statistical Manual of Mental Disorders, Third Edition*. Washington, DC: American Psychiatric Association, 1980.

Appelbaum, PS and LH Roth: Clinical Issues in the Assessment of Competency. *American J. Psychiatry* v 138:1462-1467, Nov 1981.

Auchincloss, E., and R. Michels: Psychoanalytic theory of character, in *Current Perspectives on Personality Disorders*. Edited by J. Frosch. Washington, DC: American Psychiatric Press, 1983.

Bai, Koichi: Patients' autonomy in Japan viewed in terms of consent. ACTA, Sixth World Congress on Medical Law. Gent, August 22–26, 1982, Deel 2, pp. 7–11.

Ballantine, H. Thomas, Jr.: Annual discourse—the crisis in ethics, anno domini 1979. *New England Journal of Medicine* 301:634, 1979.

Barsch, David P.: *Sociobiology and Behavior*. New York: Elsevier, 1977.

Barton, Walter, and Gail M. Barton: *Ethics and Law in Mental Health Administration*. New York: International Universities Press, 1984.

Baudry, F.: The evolution of the concept of character in Freud's writings. *Journal of the American Psychoanalytic Association* 31:1, 1983.

Beauchamp, Thomas, and James Childress: *Principles of Biomedical Ethics*. New York: Oxford University Press, 1979.

Benedict, Ruth: *Patterns of Culture*. New York: New American Library, 1958.

Berlant, Jeffrey: *Profession and Monopoly: A Study of Medicine in the United States and Great Britain*. Berkeley: University of California Press, 1975.

Bloch, Sidney, and Paul Chodoff: *Psychiatric Ethics*. New York: Oxford University Press, 1981.

Bok, Sissela: *Lying: Moral Choice in Public and Private Life*. New York: Pantheon Books, 1978.

Breuer, Joseph, and Sigmund Freud: *Studies on Hysteria* (1893–1895), pp. 143–144. Quoted in Szasz, Thomas: *The Myth of Mental Illness*. New York: Harper and Row, 1974, p. 73

Brody, Howard: *Ethical Decisions in Medicine*, 2nd ed. Boston: Little, Brown, 1981.

Budd, Louis: Altruism arrives in America. *American Quarterly* 8:40–52, Spring 1956.

Campbell, Dennis: *Doctors, Lawyers, Ministers*. Nashville: Abingdon, 1982.

Campbell, Donald: On the conflicts between biological and social evolution and between psychology and moral tradition. *American Psychologist* 30:1103–1126, 1975.

Carrick, Paul: *Medical Ethics in Antiquity*. Boston: D. Reidel, 1985.

Chapman, Carlton, B.: *Physicians, Law, and Ethics*. New York: New York University Press, 1984.

Christians C. G., Q. J. Schultze, and N. H. Simms: Community epistemology and mass media ethics. *Journalism History* 5:38–41, 65–67, 1978.

Churchill, Larry: Bioethical reductionism and our sense of the human. *Man and Medicine* 5(4):229–242, 1980.

Clouser, K. Danner: What is medical ethics? *Annals of Internal Medicine* 80:657–660, 1970.

Comte, Auguste: *System of Public Polity, 1851–1854,* 4 vols. London: Green and Company, 1875–1877.

Crimm, Allan, and Raymond Greenberg: Reflections on the doctor-patient relationship: paternalism and autonomy, in *Ethical Dimensions of Clinical Medicine*. Edited by Allen R. Dyer and Dennis R. Robbins. Springfield, IL: Charles Thomas Publishers, 1981.

Dawkins, Gerald: *The Selfish Gene.* New York: Oxford, 1976.

Dostoevsky, Fyodor: *The Brothers Karamazov.* Cited in Edel, Abraham: *Ethical Judgment: The Use of Science in Ethics.* New York: The Free Press, 1964.

Durham Morning Herald, 12 February 1986, p. 1.

Dyer, Allen R.: Can informed consent be obtained from a psychiatric patient? Reflections on the doctor-patient relationship, in *Controversy in Psychiatry*. Edited by John Paul Brady and H. Keith H. Brodie. Philadelphia: Saunders, 1978.

Dyer, Allen R.: R. D. Laing in post-critical perspective. *British Journal of Psychiatry* 124:252–259, March 1974.

Dyer, Allen R., and William B. Bunn: Natural death in medical practice. *North Carolina Medical Journal* 41:147–151, 1980.

Dyer, Allen R.: Informed consent and the non-autonomous person. *IRB: A Review of Human Subjects Research* 4:1–4, 1982.

Dyer, Allen R.: Ethics, advertising, and the definition of a profession. *Journal of Medical Ethics* 11:72–78, 1985.

Dyer, Allen R.: Assessment of competence to give informed consent, in *Senile Dementias of the Alzheimer's Type and Related Diseases: Ethical and Legal Issues Related to Informed Consent*. Edited by Vijaya L. Melnick. Clifton, NJ: Humana Press, 1985, pp. 227–237.

Dyer, Allen R.: Virtue and medicine: a physician's analysis, in *Virtue and Medicine*. Edited by Earl Shelp. Dordrecht: D. Reidel, 1985, pp. 223–235.

Dyer, Allen R.: The concept of character: moral and therapeutic considerations. *British Journal of Medical Psychology* 59:35–41, 1986.

Dyer, Allen R.: The dreams of Descartes: notes on the origins of scientific thinking. *Annual of Psychoanalysis* 14:163–175, 1986.

Dyer, Allen R., and Sidney Bloch: Informed consent and the psychiatric patient. *Journal of Medical Ethics.* 13(1):12–16, 1987.

Dyer, Susan K.: *Plinlimmon's Theme: The Aspirations and Limitations of Man in the Novels of Herman Melville*. Ph.D. thesis. Durham, NC: Duke University, 1977.

Edel, Abraham: *Ethical Judgment: The Use of Science in Ethics.* New York: The Free Press, 1964.

Edelstein, Ludwig: The Hippocratic Oath. Text, translation, and interpretation. *Bulletin of the History of Medicine* (Supplement no. 1), 1943.

Edelstein, Ludwig: *Ancient Medicine.* Baltimore: Johns Hopkins University Press, 1967.

Eisenberg, Leon: Disease and illness; distinctions between professional and popular ideas of sickness. *Culture, Medicine and Psychiatry* 1:9–23, 1977.

Engel, George: The need for a new medical model: a challenge for biomedicine. *Science* 196:129–136, 1977.

Engelhardt, H. Tristram, Jr.: The disease of masturbation: values and the concept of disease. *Bulletin of Historical Medicine* 48:234–248, 1974.

Erikson, Erik H.: *Insight and Responsibility*. New York: Norton, 1964.

Erikson, Erik H.: *Identity, Youth and Crisis*. New York: Norton, 1968.

Erikson, Erik H.: *Identity and the Lifecycle*. Psychological Issues Monograph Series, vol. 1, no. 1. New York: International Universities Press, 1959.

Everstine, Louis, and Diana Sullivan Everstine: *Psychotherapy and the Law*. Orlando, FL: Grune and Stratton, 1986.

Fletcher, Joseph: *Situation Ethics*. Philadelphia: Westminister Press, 1966.

Fletcher, Joseph: *Morals and Medicine*. Princeton: Princeton University Press, 1954.

Frankena, William: Pritchard and the ethics of virtue. *The Monist* 54:17, 1970.

Frankena, William: *Ethics*. Englewood Cliffs, NJ: Prentice-Hall, 1963.

Freedman, Daniel X. Cited in Romano, J.: Reflections on informed consent. *Archives of General Psychiatry* 30:192–235, 1974.

Freud, Sigmund: On narcissism: an introduction (1914–1916), in *The Complete Psychological Works of Sigmund Freud, Standard Edition*, vol. 14. Translated and edited by James Strachey. London: The Hogarth Press and the Institute of Psycho-Analysis, 1957.

Freud: Intepretation of dreams (1900), in *Standard Edition*, vol. 4, 1957.

Freud: Freud's psychoanalytic procedure (1904), in *Standard Edtion*, vol. 7, 1957.

Freud: Three essays on the theory of sexuality (1905), in *Standard Edition*, vol. 7, 1957.

Freud: Character and anal erotism (1908), in *Standard Edition*, vol. 9, 1957.

Freud: The disposition to obsessional neurosis (1913), in *Standard Edition*, vol. 12, 1957.

Freud: Some character types met with in psychoanalytic work (1915), in *Standard Edition*, vol. 14, 1957.

Freud: Neurosis and psychosis (1924), in *Standard Edition*, vol. 19, 1957.

Freud: Neurosis and psychosis (1930), in *Standard Edition*, vol. 21, 1957.

Freud: Civilization and its discontents (1930), in *Standard Edition*, vol. 21, 1957.

Freud: The ego and the id (1923–25), in *Standard Edition*, vol. 19, 1957.

Freud: Totem and taboo (1913–14), in *Standard Edition*, vol. 13, 1957.

Freud: Group psychology and the analysis of the ego (1921), in *Standard Edition*.

Friedson, E.: *Profession of Medicine: A Study of the Sociology of Applied Knowledge*. New York: Dodd, Mead, 1970.

Fromm: Erich: *Man for Himself: An Inquiry into the Psychology of Ethics*. New York: Holt, Rinehart, and Winston, 1947.

Furer, M.: The history of the superego concept in psychoanalysis: a review of the literature, in *Moral Values and the Superego Concept in Psychoanalysis*. Edited by Seymour C. Post. New York: International Universities Press, 1972.

Ghiselin, M.T.: *The Economy of Nature and the Evolution of Sex*. Berkeley: University of California Press, 1974.

Gilligan, James: Beyond morality: psychoanalytic reflections on shame, guilt and love. in *Moral Development and Behavior: Theory, Research, and Social*

Issues. Edited by Thomas Likona. New York: Holt, Rinehart and Winston, 1976.

Girouard, M.: *The Public Schools in the Return to Camelot: Chivalry and the English Gentlemen*. New Haven and London: Yale University Press, 1981.

Glover, E.: *War, Sadism, and Pacifism*. London: George Allen and Unwin, Ltd. 1933.

Gray B. H.: Complexities of informed consent. *Annals of the American Academy of Political Science* 437:37–48, 1978.

Greenhouse, J.: Justices uphold right of doctors to solicit trade. *The New York Times*, 24 March 1982, p. 10.

Guttentag, Otto E.: The attending physician as a central figure, in *Changing Values in Medicine*. Edited by Eric J. Cassell and Mark Siegler. Chicago: University Publications of America, 1979, pp. 107–126.

Guttentag, Otto E.: Ethical problems in human experimentation, in *Ethical Issues in Medicine*. Edited by E. F. Torrey. Boston: Little, Brown, 1968, pp. 197–226.

Guttentag, Otto E.: On defining medicine. *The Christian Scholar* 46:200–211, 1963.

Guttentag, Otto E.: The problem of experimentation on human beings: the physician's point of view. *Science* 117:205, 1953.

Hamilton, Edith: *Mythology*. Boston: Little Brown, 1942.

Hartmann, Heinz, and Rudolph Lowenstein: Notes on the superego. *Psychoanalytic Study of the Child* 17:1, 1962.

Haskell, T. L.: *The Emergence of Professional Social Science*. Urbana: University of Illinois Press, 1977.

Hauerwas, Stanley: *Community and Character*. Notre Dame: University of Notre Dame Press, 1981.

Hauerwas, Stanley: *Truthfulness and Tragedy: Further Investigation into Christian Ethics*. Notre Dame: University of Notre Dame Press, 1977.

Havighurst, Clark: Antitrust enforcement in the medical services industry: what does it all mean? *Milbank Memorial Fund Quarterly/Health and Society* 58(1):89–124, 1980.

Heyman, Gary M.: Mandated child abuse reporting and the confidentiality privilege, in *Psychotherapy and the Law*. Edited by Louis Everstine and Diana Sullivan Everstine. Orlando, FL: Grune and Stratton, 1986, pp. 145–155.

Houpt, J., C. Orleans, L. George, and H. K. H. Brodie: *The Importance of Mental Health Services for General Health Care*. Cambridge, MA: Ballinger Press, 1979.

Illych, Ivan: *Medical Nemesis*. New York: Pantheon Books, 1976.

Kant, Immanuel: *Fundamental Principles of the Metaphysic of Morals*. Indianapolis: The Library of Liberal Arts, Bobbs-Merill, 1949.

Kaplan, A.: Freud and modern philosophy, in *Freud and the 20th Century*. Edited by B. Nelson. New York: Meridian Books, 1957.

Kaplan, J., and T. Plaut: *Personality in a Communal Society*. Lawrence: University of Kansas, 1956.

Kass, Leon: Is there a medical ethic?: the Hippocratic Oath and the sources of ethical medicine, in *Toward a More Natural Science: Biology and Human Affairs*. New York: The Free Press, 1985.

Kernberg, Otto: *Borderline Conditions and Pathological Narcissism*. New York: Jason Aronson, 1971.

Kohut, Heinz: *The Analysis of the Self*. New York: International Universities Press, 1971.

Konold, Donald: Codes of medical ethics, in *Encyclopedia of Medical Ethics*, vol. 1. New York: The Free Press, 1978, pp. 162–171.

La Vopa, Anthony J.: Humanism and professional education: Historical background, in *The Humanities and the Profession of Medicine*. Edited by Allen R. Dyer. Research Triangle Park, NC: National Humanities Center, 1982, pp. 1–23.

Larson, M. S.: *The Rise of Professionalism: A Sociological Analysis*. Berkeley: University of California Press, 1977.

Lasch, Christopher: *The Culture of Narcissism: American Life in an Age of Diminishing Expectations*. New York: Norton, 1978.

Leake, Chauncey: *Percival's Medical Ethics*. Baltimore: Williams & Wilkins, 1927.

Lebacqz, Karen, and Robert J. Levine: Respect for persons and informed consent to participate in research. *Clinical Research*, vol. 25, 1977.

Lee, R. E.: Application of antitrust laws to the professions. *Journal of Legal Medicine* 1(2):143–153, 1979.

Levine, Maurice: *Psychiatry & Ethics*. New York: George Braziller, 1972.

Likona, Thomas: *Moral Development and Behavior: Theory, Research, and Social Issues*. New York: Holt, Rinehart and Winston, 1976.

Macmurray, John: *The Self as Agent*. London: Faber, 1957.

Mahler, Margaret, S., Fred Pine, and Anni Bergman: *The Psychological Birth of the Human Infant: Symbiosis and Individuation*. New York: Philosophical Library, 1944.

Maugham, Somerset: Points of view. Quoted in Castelnuovo-Tedesco, Pietro: "The mind as a stage." Some comments on reminiscence and internal objects. *International Journal of Psychoanalysis* 59:19, 1978.

Mead, Margaret: Personal communication to Maurice Levine, 1961. Quoted in Levine, Maurice: *Psychiatry & Ethics*. New York: Holt, Rinehart and Winston, 1976.

Menninger, Karl: *Whatever Became of Sin?* New York: Hawthorn, 1973.

Merleau-Ponty, Maurice: *Phenomenology of Perception*. London: Routledge and Kegan-Paul, 1962.

Michels, Robert: Professional ethics and social value. *International Review of Psychoanalysis* 3:377–384, 1976.

Mills, M. J., L. C. Hsu, and P. A. Berger: Informed consent: psychotic patients and research. *Bulletin of the American Academy of Psychiatry and the Law* 8:119–132, 1980.

Moline, Jon: On professionals and professions, in *The Humanities and the Profession of Medical Research*. Edited by Allen R. Dyer. Research Triangle Park, NC: National Humanities Center, 1982, pp. 45–65.

Moore, Charles B: This is medical ethics? *The Hastings Center Report*, November 4(5):1–3, 1974.

Mullins, Phil, and Douglas Adams: Conscience, tacit knowledge, and the art of judgment: implications of Polanyi's thought for moral reflection. *Soundings* 66(1):34–45, 1983.

Nader, Ralph, and Sidney Wolfe: Is the American health system bad for America's health? *Practical Psychology for Physicians*, December 1976, pp. 30–38.

Niebuhr, H. Richard: *The Responsible Self: An Essay in Christian Moral Philosophy*. New York: Harper and Row, 1963.

Percy, Walker: The diagnostic novel. *Harper's Magazine*, June 1986, pp. 39–45.

Pertschuk, Michael: FTC Conference, June 1-2, 1977. Quoted in Rosoff, A. J.: Antitrust laws and the health care industry: new warriors into an old battle. *Saint Louis University Law Journal* 23:478, 1979. Also quoted in Ballantine, H. Thomas, Jr.: Annual discourse—the crisis in ethics, anno domini 1979. *New England Journal of Medicine* 301:634, 1979.

Piaget, Jean: La Representation du monde chez l'enfant. Cited in Merleau-Ponty, Maurice: *Phenomenology of Perception*. London: Routledge and Kegan Paul, 1962.

Pier, G., and M. Singer: *Shame and Guilt*. Springfield, IL: Charles C Thomas, 1953.

Pincoffs, Edmund: Quandary ethics. *Mind* 75:552–571, October 1971.

Pincoffs, Edmund: Virtue, the quality of life, and punishment. *The Monist*, vol. 63, no. 2, 1980, pp. 23–27.

Polanyi, Michael: *Science, Faith and Society*. Chicago: University of Chicago Press, 1946.

Polanyi, Michael: Scientific outlook: its sickness and cure. *Science* 125:480–484, 1957.

Polanyi, Michael: *Personal Knowledge: Towards a Post-Critical Philosophy*. New York: Harper and Row, 1964.

Polanyi, Michael: The message of the Hungarian revolution. *Christianity and Crisis*, 31 October 1966, pp. 240–243.

Polanyi, Michael: The message of the Hungarian revolution. *The American Scholar* 35:661–676, Autumn 1966.

Polanyi, Michael: Life transcending physics and chemistry. *Chemical and Engineering News* 45:55–66, 1967.

Polanyi, Michael: *The Tacit Dimension*. Garden City: Doubleday, 1967.

Post, Seymour G.: Parisian masters as a corporation, 1200–1246. *Spectrum* 9:421–425, 1934.

Post, Seymour G.: *Moral Values and the Superego Concept in Psychoanalysis*. New York: International Universities Press, 1972.

Poteat, William: *Polanyian Meditations*. Durham, NC: Duke University Press, 1986.

Principles of Medical Ethics with Annotations Applicable to Psychiatry. Washington, DC: American Psychiatric Press, 1986.

Raleigh News and Observer, 13 February 1986, p. 1C.

Redlich, Fritz, and Richard Mollica: Overview: ethical issues in contemporary psychiatry. *American Journal of Psychiatry* 133(2):125–136, 1976.

Reiser, Stanley J., Arthur J. Dyck, and William J. Curran: *Ethics in Medicine: Historical Perspectives and Contemporary Concerns*. Cambridge: MIT Press, 1977.

Reich, Warren: *Character Analysis*. London: Vision Press, 1949

Relman, Arthur S.: Professional directories—but not commercial advertising—as a public service. *New England Journal of Medicine* 299:476–478, 1978.

Riskin, L.: Informed consent: looking for the action. *University of Illinois Law Forum* 4:580–611, 1975.

Robbins, Dennis A., and Allen R. Dyer: *Ethical Dimensions of Clinical Medicine*. Springfield, IL: Charles C Thomas, 1981.

Rogers, William R.: Helplessness and agency in the healing process, in *Nourishing the Humanistic in Medicine: Interactions with the Social Sciences*. Edited by William R. Rogers and David Bernard. Pittsburgh: University of Pittsburgh Press, 1979.

Romano, John: Reflections on informed consent. *Archives of General Psychiatry* 30:192–235, 1974.

Ryle, Gilbert: *The Concept of Mind*. London: Hutchison, 1949.

Schultze, Quentin J.: Professionalism in advertising: the origin of ethical codes. *Journal of Communication* 31:64–71, 1981.

Scriven, Michael: *The Science of Ethics*. Quoted in Campbell, Donald: Response to Dyer. *American Psychologist* 33:770–772, August 1978.

Sider, Roger C., and Colleen Clements: Psychiatry's contribution to medical ethics education. *American Journal of Psychiatry* 139(4):498–501, 1982.

Smith, Harmon L., and Larry Churchill: *Professional Ethics and Primary Care Medicine*. Durham, NC: Duke University Press, 1986.

Snow, C. P.: *The Two Cultures: And a Second Look; An Expanded Version of the Two Cultures and the Scientific Revolution*. Cambridge: Cambridge University Press, 1964.

Stanley, B. H., and M. Stanley: Psychiatric patients in research: protecting their autonomy. *Comprehensive Psychiatry* 22:420–427, 1981.

Strong, Carson: Informed consent: theory and practice. *Journal of Medical Ethics* 5:196–199, 1979.

Szasz, Thomas: *The Myth of Mental Illness*. New York: Harper and Row, 1974.

Tarasoff v. Regents of University of Cal., 17 Cal. 3d 425 (1976).

Thomas Arnold. *Encyclopaedia Britannica*, vol. 2, 1951.

Thrupp, S. L.: *The Guilds, Cambridge Economic History of Europe*. Cambridge: Cambridge University Press, 1963.

Tillich, Paul: *Love, Power and Justice: Ontological Analyses and Ethical Applications*. New York: Oxford University Press, 1954.

Tillich, Paul: *Systematic Theology*. Chicago: University of Chicago Press, 1951–1963.

Toennies, F.: *Fundamental Concepts of Sociology*. Translated by Charles Loomis. New York: America Book Company, 1940.

Veatch, Robert: Three theories of informed consent: philosophical foundations and policy implications. The National Commission for the Protection of Human Subjects of Biomedical and Behavioral Research (The Belmont Report), 1976.

Veatch, Robert: *A Theory of Medical Ethics*. New York: Basic Books, 1981.

Veatch, Robert: The generalization of expertise. *The Hastings Center Studies* 1:29–40, 1973.

Veatch, Robert: The Medical model: its nature and problems. *The Hastings Center Studies* 3:59–76, 1973.

Weber, Max: *On the Methodology of the Social Sciences*. Translated and edited by E. A. Shils and H. A. Finch. Glencoe: The Free Press, 1949.

Wilensky, H.: The professionalization of everyone? *The American Journal of Sociology* 70:137ff, 1964.

Wilson, E. O.: *Sociobiology: The New Synthesis*. Cambridge: Belknap/Harvard University Press, 1975.

Winslade, William J., and Judith W. Ross: Privacy, confidentiality, and autonomy in psychotherapy. *Nebraska Law Review* 64(4):497–533, 1985.

Zerubavel, E.: The bureaucratization of responsibility: the case of informed consent. *Bulletin of the American Academy of Psychiatry and the Law* 8:161–167, 1980.

Index

Abortion, 2, 32, 35, 37, 57, 73, 109
Abraham, Karl, 103, 105
Act-utilitarians, 49, 50
Adams, Douglas, 3
Adikie, 34
Advertising
  AMA code of ethics, 7, 11, 21
  codes of ethics, 20-22
  ethics of advertising, 23-26
  "right to advertise," 9
Aesculapius, 30, 32, 36, 47
Affect, 114
Agape, 49
Altruism, 13, 128-135
Amae, 142
Ambiguity
  doctor-patient relationship, 90
  in medicine, 146
  moral, in psychiatry, 10, 90
  narcissism, 133
Ambivalence, 15, 16, 50, 88-89, 123
American Medical Association
  code of ethics, 7, 11, 20, 21-22,
    33, 35, 46, 108, 109
  ethics of advertising, 23-24
  expulsion of members, 107
  FTC lawsuit, 7, 11

professional identity and
  altruism, 129
Anthropological medical
  model, 10, 72
Antipsychiatry, 125
Antisocial cults, 133
Antitrust challenge to
  professions, 22
Applebaum, Paul, 85, 91
Aristotelian, 30, 101
Aristotle, 46, 49
Arnold, Thomas, 101
Auchincloss, E., 104
Augustine, 49
Australia, 9
Authoritarian personality, 106
Authority
  Charcot's, 77
  church, 71
  criteria for exercising, 18
  decision-making, 13
  and deontological ethical
    method, 51
  ethics committee of the São
    Paulo Medical Society, 97
  government, 39
  moral, alienation of, 7

Autoeroticism, 119
Autonomy, 83-88, 97-98
    anal character, 103
    confrontation of character
        pathology, 105
    definition, 84
    dependency, 123
    medical model, 9
    versus paternalism, 13, 36-38, 91,
        93, 94, 139, 141-142

Bacon, Sir Francis, 3, 100
Beauchamp, Thomas, 85
Behavioral science, moral inversion
    and, 125
Belgium, 22, 47
Benedict, Ruth, 122
Beneficence, 8, 49, 98
Bentham, Jeremy, 49
Berlant, Jeffrey, 20
Bioethics, 5, 99, 108, 110
Biological medical model,
    2, 10, 72, 76
Bok, Sissela, 80-81
British Medical Association, 22, 60
British Medical Journal, 69
Budd, Louis, 130

Campbell, Donald, 132
Canadian Medical Association, 22
Cancer, 31, 81, 95, 140
Canterbury Tales, 17
Capital punishment, 39
Carrick, Paul, 40
Cartesian dualism, 3, 71-72, 76,
    81-82, 100
Case reports, 63
Categorical imperative, 51, 104
Chapman, Carlton, 35
Character
    and ethical decisions, 69
    in ethics, 99-107
    Japanese, 142
    judgment, 114
    in our lives, 133
    professional, 21
Character disorders, 104-106

Character ethics, 3, 99
Charaka Samhita, 30
Charcot, J. M., 77
Chaucer, Geoffrey, 17
Child abuse reporting, 66
Childress, James, 85
Christianity, 30, 122, 129
Clements, Colleen, 99
Clinical judgment, 5, 6, 70, 80, 113,
    114
Clouser, K. Danner, 46
Codes of ethics, 12
    advertising, 22
    American Medical Association, 7,
        21, 27
    British, Belgian, Canadian, 22
    Charaka Samhita, 30
    Percival's code, 20
    World Medical Association, 22
Cogito, 112, 117
Commitment (civil)
    opposition as moral inversion,
        124
    Szasz's criticism, 77, 79-80
    Tarasoff decision, 61
Commitment (personal)
    definition of a profession, 15, 16,
        106
    double agentry, 68
    Hippocratic, 66, 96
    to the individual versus the
        group, 65
Competence assessment, 85-86
Comte, Auguste, 129
Confidence
    crisis of, 9, 56, 93
    informed consent in England, 92
    narcissistic syndrome, 133
    principle of partnership, 87
    public, 18, 108-109
    sexual contact as violation, 33
    See also Confidentiality
Confidentiality
    case reports, 63
    child abuse reporting, 66
    codes of ethics, 59
    conflicts, 60
    cost containment and, 63

custody case testimony, 66
definition of a profession, 17, 32
essential virtue of the medical
  profession, 108-109
fraud prevention, 62
group therapy, 65
Hippocratic Oath, 32, 59
Hippocratic Oath for
  Psychiatrists, 43, 44
legal status, 60, 69
nonprofessional involvement in
  'health care teams, 66
patient access to records, 65
prearraignment examinations, 63
professional gossip, 64
public safety and, 61
redisclosure and, 62
therapeutic alliance, 58-70
Conflict, ethics and, 114, 126
Consent. See Informed consent
Consequentialist approach, 53-57
Cost containment
  conflict with Hippocratic Oath, 40
  physician as agent, 63
"Crisis of the personal," 117-118
Curran, William J., 17
Custody cases, 66

Darwinism, 130
Decision making
  contextual process, 112-113
  deontological ethical method, 51
  dimension of time, 91
  instantaneous act, 38
  involving a third person, 90
  medical versus ethical, 5-6
  of patient, 86
  patient's versus physician's, 94
  teleological ethical method, 49
Deontological theory of ethics, 12,
  48, 49, 51-53, 84, 121, 144
Dependency
  informed consent, 91
  mature character, 103, 123
  sexual contact with patients,
    33-34
  versus autonomy, 83-86, 141-143
De-professionalization, 4

Descartes, Réné, 3, 71, 76, 112, 123,
  145. See also Cartesian dualism
Disease, distinguished from
  illness, 74, 75
Dissemination of information, 24
Doctor-patient relationship
  confidentiality, 32, 60-61
  in definition of a profession, 5
  development over time, 144
  focus for ethical dilemmas, 82
  traditional versus contemporary
    structure, 26
  virtues of the patient, 109
  See also Autonomy; Paternalism
Doi, Takeo, 142
Donaldson, Sir John, 93
Dostoevsky, Fyodor, 112, 124
Double agent problem, 68
Downwards perspective, 48, 65,
  111, 121
Dualism. See Cartesian dualism
Duty
  breach of, 92
  in Campbell's characterization of
    psychology and psychiatry, 132
  defining deontological
    functioning, 51
  to delivery health care equitably,
    34
  of society to protect physicians,
    31
  to warn, 61
Dyck, Arthur J., 17
Dynamo-objective coupling, 125

Economic aspects of professions,
  15, 18. See also Advertising
Ego, 13, 102, 119-122, 134
Engel, George, 10, 76
Engelhardt, H. Tristam, 134
Enlightenment, 3, 4, 8, 111, 139
Epidemiology, 143
Epistemology
  Cartesian, 76
  distinguished from ethical
    problems, 81, 112
  moral inversion, 123-124
  Polanyi's, 117, 124, 145

sterility of, 100
in Szasz's criticism of Freud, 78
Erikson, Erik H., 84
Ethical codes. *See* Codes of ethics
Ethical theories, 12, 49-50, 51, 52,
    121, 144
Ethics
    advertising issues, 23-24, 26
    concept of virtue, 107
    conflicts, 10
    consequentialist, 53, 54
    decision making, 6, 113-115
    definition, 45-49
    legal perspectives, 69-70
    perspectives on, 48
    psychiatry's dilemmas, 10
    responsibility, 137-147
    role in professional conduct, 15
    science as basis for, 56
    See also Medical ethics
Ethicist, 5, 6, 114, 115, 140
Euthanasia, 2, 32, 35, 37, 50
Expertise, 4-7, 17-18, 107, 137, 139

Fawkes, Guy, 60
Federal Trade Commission v.
    American Medical Association
    and others, 7, 11, 23
Fiduciary nature of doctor-patient
    relationship, 5, 12, 47, 48, 70,
    80, 90, 91, 124, 146
Fletcher, Joseph, 49
Frankena, William, 49, 55
Fraud prevention, 62
Freeman v. Home Office, 92-93
Freud, Sigmund, 77-79, 100-104,
    118-120, 130
Fromm, Erich, 101

Gatekeeping function of
    professional organizations,
    106-108
Gemeinschaft, 45, 47
Geneva, Declaration of, 39, 59, 91,
    94-95
Gesellschaft, 45, 47
Ghana, 47

Gilligan, James, 121, 122
Girouard, Mark, 101
God, 51, 56, 118, 123, 141, 145
Goldfarb decision, 22
Goldwater, Barry, 64
Gossip of professionals, 64
Gothenburg, Sweden, 94
Great Britain, 34, 91, 92
Grief, 144
Group therapy, 65
Guilt
    character, 101
    in moral vocabulary, 129
    regulator of morality, 121-123
Gunpowder plot, 60
Guttentag, Otto E., 10, 72, 73, 87
Guyana, 133

Happiness, 49, 50, 51, 53
Hartman, Heinz, 120
Hastings Center, 46
Hauerwas, Stanley, 55, 112, 117, 145
Health maintenance organization,
    68
Health services distribution, 34
Heisenberg Uncertainty Principle, 4
Hippocratic Oath, 41
    abortion, 32
    advertising, 20-21
    confidentiality, 59-60
    criticisms of, 34-36
    defense of, 36-38
    distribution of health services, 34
    euthanasia, 32
    Hippocratic tradition, 29-30, 31,
        33, 34-37, 40
    history and significance, 29-31
    patient benefit, 34
    patient confidentiality, 32
    professional affiliations, 34
    relevance, 35, 36, 40
    sexual contact with patients, 33
    truth-telling, 33
    trustworthiness, 108
    See also Hippocratic tradition
Hippocratic Oath for Psychiatrists,
    42-44
Hippocratic tradition, 29-44

behind the Iron Curtain, 96
role in modern medicine, 139
trust as characteristic, 9
See also Hippocratic Oath
Homosexuality, 73, 75, 109
Human rights, 39, 91, 125-126
Humane understanding, 2
Hypochondria, 73
Hysteria, 77-78

Idealism in medical ethics, 13,
    111, 119-121, 123, 124, 134, 146
Idealized parent, 120
Illness, distinguished from
    disease, 74, 75
Illych, Ivan, 71
Impersonality of medicine, 137
Infantilizing, 86
Informed consent, 83-98
    autonomy principle, 84
    case reports, 64
    competence, 85-86
    definition, 86-87
    disclosure in information banks,
        63
    in Great Britain, 91-93
    in Iron Curtain countries, 96
    in Japan and Asian Pacific, 95
    medical ethics, 139
    medical model, 9
    medical responsibility, 140
    partnership principle, 87-89
    process, 89-91
    review of Medicare records, 62
    in Sweden, 94
    torture, 96-97
    in United States, 140
Institutional Review Board, 48
Integrity
    character, 102
    in ethical decision making, 113
    inhibitory moral traditions, 134
    hallmark of moral life, 55, 112
    in Hippocratic Oath for
        Psychiatrists, 44
    moral, 13, 40, 47
    psychosomatic, 82

scientific, 139
Involuntary hospitalization, 62,
    78-80

Judgment. *See* Clinical judgment
Justice, 34, 51, 115, 125

Kant, Immanuel, 51, 84, 122
Kaplan, Abraham, 105
Kaplan, J., 122
Karamazov, Ivan, 112
Kohut, Heinz, 135
Kwakiutl Indians, 122

Lafcadio, 124
Lasch, Christopher, 129
Leake, Chauncey, 35, 46, 72
Legal perspectives on ethics, 69-70
Lethal injections, 32, 40
Levine, Maurice, 12, 42-44
Lifestyle, 31, 36
Lowenstein, Rudolph, 120
Loyalty, 51, 90, 109

Macmurray, John, 115, 117-118, 145
Mandatory reporting, 66, 68
Marketplace, 7-9, 17, 23
Marxism, 125, 126, 138
Maturity, 103
Maugham, Somerset, 116
Mead, Margaret, 30
Medical ethics
    advertising, 7, 11, 21, 23-24, 26
    autonomy vs. paternalism,
        139-141
    character and virtue, 99
    definition, 45-49
    education, 99
    examples, 47
    idealism, 13, 119-121, 123, 124,
        146
    impersonality, 5, 7
    informed consent, 140
    morality, 46
    responsibility, 145
    role, 72

virtue in gatekeeping
function, 107
Medical etiquette, 46, 72
Medical model
ambiguity of, 72
anthropological, 10, 72, 144, 147
biological, 10, 72, 76, 144, 147
confidentiality, 60
psychiatry and, 9-11
Medicine
definition, 73-76
as profession, 16-18
as science, 137-138
as technology, 4, 7, 71
as trade, 11, 23, 25, 27
Menninger, Karl, 132-133
Mental Health Act 1983 (Great
Britain), 92, 93, 104
Mental illness, viewed as myth,
76-77
Merleau-Ponty, Maurice, 116-117
Michels, Robert, 104
Mill, John Stuart, 49, 84
Mind-body problem, 12, 71, 73, 80,
82
Mollica, Richard, 83
Monopoly, 15, 17, 18, 20, 23
Moore, Charles, 46
Moore, G. E., 49
Moral ideal, 7, 13, 79
Moral imperative, 13, 48, 79, 134
Moral inversion, 79, 106, 123-126,
133
Moral perfection, 79, 111, 131
Morality
character and psychotherapy,
100, 103
as destructive force, 123
Hippocratic Oath, 30
moral tradition, 131-132, 134
sense of agency, 122
shame and guilt as regulators,
121-123
Moral self, 118-121
Mowrer, O. H., 132, 133
Mullins, Phil, 3
Myth of mental illness, 76, 77

Nader, Ralph, 71
Narcissism, 119, 120, 122, 129,
133-135
Naturalistic healing, 31
Nicomachean ethics, 46
Niebuhr, H. Richard, 144-145
Nietzsche, Friedrich, 122
Noncompliant patients, 142-143,
144
Nonprofessionals on health care
teams, 66
Nuremberg, 39, 93

Obedience, 21, 51, 103
Obligation. See Duty
L'Ordre des Medicins (Belgium), 22
Osler, Sir William, 137-139

Partnership patient-physician, 48,
69-70, 87-89, 94, 98, 139, 141,
146
Paternalism
and Hippocratic medicine, 8, 38
approach toward patients, 83, 88,
90, 91, 139-141
Berlant's view, 20
changing attitudes of patients, 36
in England, 93
in Sweden, 94
Patient benefit, 34
Patient confidentiality. See
Confidentiality
Patient virtues, 109
Patient's rights, 9, 79, 83, 84, 90,
93-96, 140, 141
Hippocratic Oath, 29, 35, 37
civil, 80
Percival, Thomas. See Percival's
code
Percival's code, 20, 21, 35, 59, 108,
109
Perfectionism, 120-126. See also
Moral perfection
Personality disorders, 104-106
Personhood, 51, 82, 84, 116, 118
Perspective, as task of ethics, 48,

111, 121
Pertschuk, Michael B., 23
Philippines, 95
Physicians
  capital punishment participation, 39
  cost containment, 40
  doctor-patient relationship, 1, 2, 5, 12, 26-27, 70, 80, 90-91
  political abuse of psychiatry, 39
  torture cooperation, 39
Piaget, Jean, 117
Pincoffs, Edmund, 55, 117
Placebos, 80-82
Plato, 49, 129
Plaut, T., 122
Pluralistic society, 45, 133-134
Poddar, Prosenjit, 61
Polanyi, M., 3, 4, 77, 106, 123-125, 131, 138, 145, 146
Political abuse of psychiatry, 39, 96
Positivism, 100, 117
Post-critical philosophy, 48, 113, 123, 124
Prearraignment examinations, 63
Principle of autonomy, 12, 83-85, 87
Privacy, in doctor-patient relationship, 11, 12, 59, 62, 63, 69, 70
Privilege, 61
Product differentiation, 24
Professions
  affiliations in Hippocratic medicine, 31, 34
  checklist, 16
  criteria, 17, 18, 25
  definition, 4, 15, 16
  ethics, 47
  professionalization, 19
  professional organizations, 31, 106-107
Psychiatry
  biological medical model, 2, 9, 76
  divided profession, 1
  Hippocratic Oath, 42-44
  moral inversion, 125
  partnership principle of psychotherapy, 88

political abuse, 39
prohibition of sexual contact with patients, 33
Psychoanalysis
  theory of character, 102
  treatment of character disorders, 104-106
Psychohistory, 64
Public safety vs. confidentiality, 61

Quandary ethics, 3
Quinlan, Karen, 49, 114, 115

Rational development, 116-117
Records, access by patients, 63
Redlich, Fritz, 83
Reich, Wilhelm, 103
Reiser, Stanley J., 17
Relativism, 56
Resistance, 102-103
Responsibility
  doctors', 6, 8, 11, 13, 137-147
  patients', 109
Restraint of trade, 7, 11, 23
Right to advertise, 9
Right to choose, 32
Right to life, 32
Rights. See Human rights; Patients' rights; Right to advertise; Right to choose, Right to life
Roe v. Wade, 37
Roth, Loren, 85, 91
Rule-utilitarians, 49
Ryle, Gilbert, 118

Schizophrenia, 79, 88, 96
Science
  as basis for ethics, 56
  value-neutral, 138
Scriven, Michael, 56
Self
  as moral agent, 111-112
  moral self, 118-121
  personhood, 116-117
Self-determination, 12, 83-85, 137, 139

Sexual contact with patients, 33
Shame, 75, 84, 101, 106, 121-123
Sherman Anti-Trust Act, 7, 22
Sidaway v. Bethlem Royal Hospital Governors, 92, 93
Sider, Roger, 99
Sin, 132
Sociobiology, 131-132
Sociological theory of professions, 15, 18
Stanley, B. H., 86
Stanley, M., 86
Suicide, 32, 35, 50, 68, 121
Superego, 13, 119-122, 134
Supreme Court, 9, 22, 23, 37, 61
Sweden, 47, 94
Szasz, Thomas, 12, 71, 76-79

Tacit knowing, 7, 48, 86, 107, 124, 125, 144
Tarasoff decision, 61-62, 66
Technology, medical ethics and, 1, 8
Teleological theories of ethics, 12, 49-50, 121, 144
Temporal thickness, 116
Therapeutic alliance, 12, 58, 59, 66, 69
Time dimension, informed consent and, 91, 141
Torture, 39, 96
Trade
  medicine as, 17, 25, 27
  psychiatry as, 2, 7
Truffaut, François, 105
Trust, in doctor-patient relationship, 33, 60, 87, 90. *See also* Confidentiality
Torture, 39, 96
Trade
  medicine as, 17, 25, 27
  psychiatry as, 2, 7

Trustworthiness
  professional criterion, 18, 20, 25
  as virtue essential to medical profession, 108
  as virtue of patients, 109
Truth-telling
  Hippocratic tradition, 33
  placebos as issue, 80-81

Uncertainty, as problem in narcissism, 133
Uncertainty Principle, 4
Upwards perspective, 48, 65, 111, 121
Utang na loob, 95
Utilitarianism. *See* Teleological theories of ethics

Value-neutral science, 138
Veatch, Robert, 6, 36
Virtue
  concept of, 99
  medical virtues, 108-109
  patients' virtues, 109-110
  in professional self-regulation, 106-108

Weber, Max, 18, 20
Wholistic medicine, 82
World Health Organization, definition of medicine, 73
World Medical Association International Code of Medical Ethics, 22
World Psychiatric Association, 39
World Medical Association International Code of Medical Ethics, 22
World Psychiatric Association, 39